THIRD EDITION

DOSAGE CALCULATION

A SIMPLIFIED APPROACH

Billie Ann Wilson, RN, MS, MN, PhD
Professor and Director
Loyola University Nursing Program
New Orleans, Louisiana

Margaret T. Shannon, RN, MS, MAT, MN, PhD
Professor and Dean
Division of Nursing
Our Lady of Holy Cross College
New Orleans, Louisiana

APPLETON & LANGE
Stamford, Connecticut

99 00 / 10 9 8 7 6 5 4 3 2

Prentice Hall International (UK) Limited, *London*
Prentice Hall of Australia, Pty. Limited, *Sydney*
Prentice Hall Canada, Inc., *Toronto*
Prentice Hall Hispanoamericana, S.A., *Mexico*
Prentice Hall of India Private Limited, *New Delhi*
Prentice Hall of Japan, Inc., *Tokyo*
Prentice Hall Asia Pte. Ltd., *Singapore*
Editora Prentice Hall do Brasil, Ltda., *Rio de Janeiro*
Prentice Hall, *Upper Saddle River, New Jersey*

Library of Congress Cataloging-in-Publication Data

Wilson, Billie Ann.
    Dosage calculation: a simplified approach / Billie Ann Wilson,
Margaret T. Shannon.—3rd ed.
        p.   cm.
    Rev. ed. of: A unified approach to dosage calculations / Billie
Ann Wilson, Margaret T. Shannon. 2nd ed. © 1991
    ISBN 0-8385-9297-X (pbk.: alk. paper)
    1. Pharmaceutical arithmetic. 2. Nursing—Mathematics.
I. Shannon, Margaret T.   II. Wilson, Billie Ann. Unified approach to
dosage calculations.   III. Title.
    [DNLM: 1. Drugs—administration & dosage—problems. 2. Drugs—
administration & dosage—nurses' instruction. 3. Mathematics—
problems. 4. Mathematics—nurses' instruction.   QV 18.2 W746d
1996]
RS57.W55   1996
615'.14'01513—dc20
DNLM/DLC   96-20502
for Library of Congress   CIP

Acquisitions Editor: Kathleen L. Riedell
Production Editor: Maria T. Vlasak
Designer: Mary Skudlarek

ISBN 0-8385-9297-X

PRINTED IN THE UNITED STATES OF AMERICA

Contents

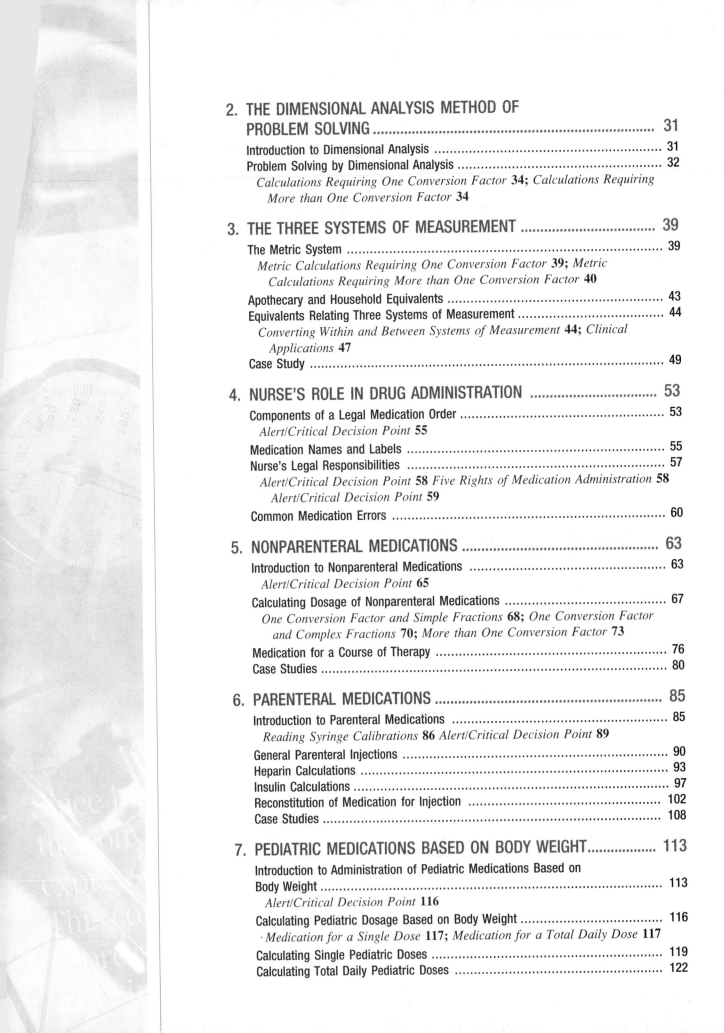

About the Authors

Billie Ann Wilson is currently the Director of the Baccalaureate Program in Nursing at Loyola University in New Orleans, Louisiana. Prior to entering nursing she taught natural and physical sciences at the secondary and collegiate levels. She holds a Bachelor of Science in Biology from Boston College, a Master of Science in Biology from Purdue University, a Bachelor of Science in Nursing from Northwestern State University of Louisiana, and a Master of Nursing from Louisiana State University Medical Center and a PhD in Curriculum and Instruction from the University of New Orleans.

Margaret T. Shannon is currently the Dean of the Baccalaureate Program in Nursing at Our Lady of Holy Cross College, New Orleans. Her educational preparation includes a Bachelor of Science in Chemistry, a Master of Science in Chemistry, both from Saint Louis University, a Master of Arts in Teaching Biology from Saint Mary's College, a Bachelor of Science in Nursing from Northwestern State University of Louisiana, a Master of Nursing from Louisiana State University Medical Center, and a PhD in Curriculum and Instruction from the University of New Orleans. Prior to entering nursing, she taught physical science, natural science, and mathematics at the secondary and collegiate levels.

Acknowledgments

Special thanks to the following pharmaceutical and health supply companies for permission to reproduce their drug labels in this text: Basel Pharmaceuticals, a Division of CIBA-GEIGY Corporation; Baxter Healthcare Corporation; Bristol Laboratories, a Division of Bristol-Meyers Company; Burroughs Wellcome Company; CIBA Pharmaceutical Co., a Division of CIBA-GEIGY Corporation; Dista Products Company, a Division of Eli Lilly Industries, Inc.; Eli Lilly and Company; Elkins-Sinn, Inc., a subsidiary of A. H. Robbins Company; Geigy Pharmaceuticals, a Division of CIBA-GEIGY Corporation; Hoechst-Roussel Pharmaceuticals, Inc.; Marion Merrel Dow, Inc.; Novo Nordisk Pharmaceuticals, Inc.; Parke-Davis, a Division of Warner-Lambert Co.; Pfizer Labs, a Division of Pfizer Inc.; Roerig, a Division of Pfizer Pharmaceuticals; and Schwarz Pharma.

To the Educator

This book is designed for students and practitioners of nursing. The format permits self-mastery of all the mathematical concepts related to drug administration presented in the text. The purpose of this book is to present a single method of problem solving that is applicable to all types of medication and intravenous fluid calculations. The text goes far beyond the usual introduction to oral and parenteral medications. It has complete coverage of *all* types of calculations related to intravenous administration of fluids and medications including: general fluid replacement; replacement of blood, blood products, and plasma expanders; and continuous and intermittent infusion of medications. The text also has a thorough coverage of drugs commonly used in critical care settings, including those administered according to μg/kg/min. In addition, it has extensive coverage of pediatric dosage calculations based on mg/kg and a complete chapter on dilution of intravenous pediatric medications. Also included in the text is a chapter on chemotherapeutic and pediatric drug dosages based on the body surface area (BSA) of the client. As newly developed drugs that are effective but potentially toxic are used, the staff nurse must know how to determine the appropriate amount of medication based on the BSA of the client.

A new chapter on the nurse's role in drug administration has also been added to this edition. In this chapter and throughout the text, references are made to the nurse's legal responsibilities with regard to drug administration.

The text contains more than five hundred dosage calculation problems, all of which represent clinically correct dosage forms and quantities; both generic and trade names are used throughout. Exercises in correctly reading drug labels are included in the majority of the chapters. Critical Decision Point scenarios, as well as case studies, are used to enhance critical thinking skills. Case studies are used in a summary fashion at the end of all chapters on dosage calculations. Case studies incorporate the use of medication labels (actual manufacturer's labels or computer printout labels) to provide the student with practice in reading such labels. Each case study contains questions and calculations designed to assess the understanding of information required in medication preparation and administration.

To further assist the student in mastering the concepts contained in this text, UNICALC, a self-paced student tutorial, has been packaged with this book. Containing approximately sixty additional exercises in dimensional analysis and dosage calculation, UNICALC is interactive and student-friendly, providing not only correct answers to exercises, but rationales for incorrect answers as well as references which are tied directly to the text. UNICALC will also track student progress through its computerized program and provide a summary of results, identifying areas requiring additional study.

The text uses a problem-solving method called dimensional analysis, also referred to as the factor-label method. Dimensional analysis builds on simple arithmetic skills and does not require the memorization of multiple formulas but, rather, the application of a single method to *all types* of drug calculations. Dimensional analysis is not a new problem-solving method since it has been widely used in science education at both the secondary and collegiate levels for almost 50 years. Dimensional analysis is a refinement of the ratio and proportion method and can be used to solve any problem involving direct proportion. This method is universally applicable to dosage calculations because all medication and intravenous fluid calculations are based on direct proportion.

The dimensional analysis method is introduced in Chapter 2 and fully developed in Chapter 3; thereafter, it is used throughout the text to solve all problems presented. Mastery of Chapter 2 and Chapter 3 is therefore essential prior to study of other chapters. Once these chapters have been mastered, the remaining chapters may be studied in a variety of sequences suitable to any particular curriculum.

Chapter 1 on prerequisite arithmetic skills for dosage calculations is provided for review. All students should complete the Prerequisite Test of Arithmetic Skills to determine possible areas of weakness. Students who need review are directed to specific sections of Chapter 1 based on their performance on the prerequisite test. Chapter 1 includes mathematical operations with Roman numerals, simple and complex fractions, mixed numbers, improper fractions, decimal numbers, and percents. Following review of Chapter 1, the student may take all or part of the Post-test of Arithmetic Skills to assure competency before beginning dosage calculations.

To the Student

This text presents a single approach to dosage calculations called dimensional analysis. You may be familiar with dimensional analysis (also referred to as the factor-label method) since it is widely used in science courses. The name dimensional analysis comes from the fact that each number used in a problem retains the label (dimension) it has in the word problem. Dimensional analysis is based on ratio and proportion and can be used to solve *any* problem involving a dosage calculation regardless of the degree of complexity of the problem.

It is much more difficult to make an error when using dimensional analysis than it is when using simple ratio and proportion. Listed below are some of the safeguards of calculating with dimensional analysis.

1. It eliminates the common error of placing a number incorrectly into the numerator or the denominator of the solved problem.
2. It provides a means of determining that all needed quantities have been included in the calculation.
3. It provides a means of accurately determining which quantities are not needed in the calculation.
4. It permits visual inspection of the problem to determine that it is set up correctly.

The textbook has many features that will aid you in the learning process. Chapter 1 on arithmetic skills needed for dosage calculations is provided for your review. You should complete the Prerequisite Test of Arithmetic Skills to determine your possible areas of weakness. If you need to review you will be directed to study specific sections of Chapter 1 based on your performance on the prerequisite test. If you do not need arithmetic review, you should proceed to Chapter 2. Following any needed review of Chapter 1, and before beginning Chapter 2, you should take all or part of the Post-test of Arithmetic Skills necessary to assess your ability to use arithmetic skills.

To further assist you in mastering the concepts contained in this text, UNICALC, a self-paced student tutorial, has been packaged with this book. Containing approximately sixty additional exercises in dimensional analysis and dosage calculation, UNICALC is interactive and student-friendly, providing not only correct answers to exercises, but rationales for incorrect answers as well as references which are tied directly to the text. UNICALC will also track your progress through its computerized program and provide a summary of results, identifying areas requiring additional study.

It is important that you read the instructional content in each chapter before trying to work the problems. Start each chapter by working through the step-by-step example at the beginning of the chapter. It introduces new concepts and illustrates the application of dimensional analysis to the problem. On completion of each chapter, work *all* the problems in the self-test. If you can successfully solve 90% of the problems on a self-test, you have mastered the content in the chapter.

Calculation errors can be avoided by carrying out all steps of a problem on paper. A misplaced decimal or an inverted fraction could mean that an incorrect medication dosage would be given. Therefore, it is important that you work each problem in the text using paper and pencil.

The text contains more than five-hundred dosage calculation problems, all of which represent clinically correct dosage forms and quantities. Both generic and trade names are used throughout the text. The role of the nurse in drug administration has been added to this edition and is discussed in Chapter 4; this includes the nurse's legal responsibilities in its regard. The legal responsibilities of the nurse are emphasized throughout the text by the user of *critical decision points* related to drug administration by various routes.

The addition to this text of colored drug labels and various syringes will enhance your ability to study actual drug labels and to understand the various calibrations on syringes. Within various solved problem sets found in the text, the correct volume of the medication has been pictorially represented with a filled syringe so that you may visualize the correct dosage.

Prerequisite Arithmetic Skills

▲ OBJECTIVES

Upon completion of Chapter 1, the student will be able to:

- ► Correctly convert between Roman numerals and Arabic numbers.
- ► Correctly reduce fractions to lowest terms.
- ► Correctly compare the magnitude of fractions.
- ► Correctly add, subtract, multiply, and divide fractions.
- ► Correctly add, subtract, multiply, and divide mixed numbers or improper fractions.
- ► Correctly compare the magnitude of decimals.
- ► Correctly add, subtract, multiply, and divide decimals.
- ► Correctly convert from fractions to decimals.
- ► Correctly multiply or divide a number by 10, 100, or 1000.
- ► Correctly simplify complex fractions.
- ► Correctly convert a decimal or a fraction to a percent.
- ► Find the percent one number is of another.

▲ PREREQUISITE TEST OF ARITHMETIC SKILLS

The prerequisite test is divided into several sections. Each section corresponds to a specific section of Chapter 1. If all of your answers to a specific section are not correct, you should review the corresponding section of Chapter 1.

Roman Numerals

1. Write the following Roman numerals as Arabic numbers.

     A. xii   B. iv   C. xxv

2. Write the Roman numeral that corresponds to each number.

    A. 6   B. 13   C. 19

Reducing Fractions

3. Reduce the following fractions to lowest terms.

    A. $\dfrac{5}{15}$ B. $\dfrac{25}{100}$ C. $\dfrac{16}{24}$

    D. $\dfrac{125}{250}$ E. $\dfrac{100}{300}$ F. $\dfrac{3}{6}$

Comparing the Magnitude of Fractions

4. Determine the larger fraction in the pair of numbers.

    A. $\dfrac{1}{16}, \dfrac{1}{32}$ B. $\dfrac{2}{3}, \dfrac{1}{6}$ C. $\dfrac{2}{4}, \dfrac{3}{8}$

5. Place the following fractions in order from lowest to highest value.

    A. $\dfrac{1}{4}, \dfrac{1}{3}, \dfrac{1}{6}$ B. $\dfrac{3}{7}, \dfrac{5}{6}, \dfrac{2}{3}$ C. $\dfrac{1}{4}, \dfrac{2}{10}, \dfrac{2}{3}$

Addition and Subtraction of Fractions

6. Add or subtract the following fractions. Express your answer in lowest terms.

    A. $\dfrac{2}{3} - \dfrac{1}{6} =$ B. $\dfrac{2}{4} - \dfrac{1}{4} =$ C. $\dfrac{3}{7} - \dfrac{5}{14} =$

    D. $\dfrac{3}{5} + \dfrac{1}{2} =$ E. $\dfrac{2}{3} + \dfrac{1}{3} =$ F. $\dfrac{1}{6} + \dfrac{3}{7} =$

Multiplication and Division of Fractions

7. Multiply or divide the following fractions. Express your answer in lowest terms.

    A. $\dfrac{1}{8} \times \dfrac{4}{3} =$ B. $\dfrac{1}{6} \times \dfrac{5}{1} \times \dfrac{1}{2} =$ C. $\dfrac{3}{9} \times \dfrac{6}{10} =$

    D. $\dfrac{2}{5} \div \dfrac{2}{10} =$ E. $\dfrac{1}{150} \div \dfrac{1}{250} =$ F. $\dfrac{1}{32} \div \dfrac{1}{64} =$

Mixed Numbers and Improper Fractions

8. Express your answer as a whole number or a mixed number in lowest terms.

    A. $1\dfrac{2}{3} + \dfrac{1}{3} =$ B. $\dfrac{2}{9} + 4\dfrac{3}{4} =$ C. $\dfrac{8}{3} - \dfrac{2}{4} =$

    D. $3\dfrac{1}{4} - 2\dfrac{1}{2} =$ E. $2\dfrac{1}{2} \div 3 =$ F. $1\dfrac{1}{4} \div \dfrac{3}{2} =$

Comparing the Magnitude of Decimals

9. Place in order from lowest to highest value.

   A. 0.3, 0.32, 0.37   B. 0.02, 0.4, 0.1   C. 0.6, 0.75, 0.35

   D. 0.009, 0.900, 0.909   E. 0.12, 0.21, 0.021   F. 0.551, 0.515, 0.155

Addition, Subtraction, Multiplication, and Division of Decimals

10. Express all answers to the nearest tenth.

    A. $4.2 + 0.35 =$ B. $7.3 - 5 =$ C. $14 \times 2.3 =$

    D. $1.52 \times 0.3 =$ E. $14.3 \div 7.1 =$ F. $0.62 \div 0.21 =$

Changing Fractions to Decimals

11. Change each of the following fractions to a decimal, and then express the answer to the nearest tenth.

    A. $\dfrac{3}{8} =$ B. $\dfrac{2}{7} =$ C. $\dfrac{2}{3} =$

    D. $\dfrac{12}{14} =$ E. $\dfrac{15}{20} =$ F. $\dfrac{5}{9} =$

Multiplication and Division by 10, 100, and 1000

12. Multiply or divide the following by moving the decimal point the appropriate number of places.

    A. $12 \times 10 =$ B. $250 \times 10 =$ C. $0.032 \times 100 =$

    D. $150 \div 100 =$ E. $\dfrac{250}{1000} =$ F. $12.5 \div 10 =$

Simplifying Complex Fractions

13. Express the final answer in a decimal rounded to the nearest tenth.

    A. $\dfrac{\frac{1}{2}}{\frac{1}{6}} =$ B. $\dfrac{\frac{1}{150}}{\frac{1}{200}} =$ C. $\dfrac{\frac{1}{4}}{\frac{1}{5}} =$

    D. $\dfrac{250}{\frac{1}{6}} =$ E. $\dfrac{\frac{0.5}{2}}{\frac{1}{4}} =$ F. $\dfrac{\frac{2}{3}}{\frac{1}{6}} =$

Changing Decimals and Fractions to Percents

14. Change the following to percents.

    A. 0.17   B. 0.09   C. 0.66

    D. $\dfrac{1}{2}$ E. $\dfrac{1}{4}$ F. $\dfrac{4}{5}$

Calculations with Percent

15. Change the following percents to a decimal.
    A. 0.85%   B. 2.3%   C. 25%

16. Multiply by the percent.
    A. What is 18% of 24?
    B. What is 6% of 16.5?
    C. What is 3.2% of 12?

17. Find the percent one number is of another.
    A. What percent of 25 is 5?
    B. What percent of 100 is 9?
    C. What percent of 50 is 10?

For answers to the prerequisite test, see page 25.

▲ ROMAN NUMERALS

Roman numerals are used in doctor's orders of medications in the apothecary system of measurement. Consequently it is important that the nursing student be able to read the Roman numerals accurately. Lowercase letters rather than uppercase letters are used. Below is a list of the first ten numerals with their Arabic equivalents:

ROMAN NUMERALS	ARABIC NUMBERS
i	1
ii	2
iii	3
iv	4
v	5
vi	6
vii	7
viii	8
ix	9
x	10

It may be observed from the above list that certain rules apply to Roman numeral values.

RULE ►

 If a numeral of lesser value follows one of greater value it is added to that numeral.

Example 1.1:

vi = 5 + 1 = 6

Example 1.2:

xvii = 10 + 5 + 1 + 1 = 17

 Numerals of the same value are repeated in sequence.

◀ RULE

Example 1.3:

xxii = 10 + 10 + 1 + 1 = 22

Example 1.4:

viii = 5 + 1 + 1 + 1 = 8

 If a numeral of lesser value precedes one of greater value it is subtracted from it.

◀ RULE

Example 1.5:

xix = 10 + 10 − 1 = 19

Example 1.6:

xiv = 10 + 5 − 1 = 14

▶ **SELF-TEST**

Write the following as Arabic numbers.

1. xiii   2. vii   3. ix

4. xxiv   5. xv

Write the Roman numerals that correspond to each number.

6. 2   7. 11   8. 16

9. 8   10. 25

For answers to the self-test, see page 27.

▲ COMMON FRACTIONS

The ability to work with fractions is necessary when carrying out drug calculations because certain medications are both ordered and dispensed in fractional quantities. Incorrect arithmetic could result in overdosing or underdosing the patient.

A fraction is a part of a whole. A pie, for example, may be divided into two parts. Each part represents one-half of the whole pie.

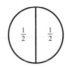

A fractional part is represented by one number divided by another. The top number is the numerator and the bottom number is the denominator. In the fraction 2/4, 2 is termed the numerator and 4 is termed the denominator.

Study the picture below. Note that 1/4 + 1/4 = 2/4, and it also equals 1/2. In fact, 1/2 represents the fraction 2/4 in its lowest term.

Reducing Fractions

In the previous diagram it was observed that 2/4 = 1/2.

RULE ▶

 A fraction may be reduced if the numerator and denominator are both evenly divisible by the same number.

Example 1.7: Reduce 2/4 to lowest terms.

Solution: Both 2 and 4 are evenly divisible by 2.

$$\frac{2}{4} = \frac{1}{2}$$

Example 1.8: Reduce 27/54 to lowest terms.

Solution: Both 27 and 54 are evenly divisible by 3, 9, and 27. However, assuming that the first number considered was 3, the resulting fraction is shown below.

$$\frac{27}{54} = \frac{9}{18}$$

Now both 9 and 18 are further divisible by 3 and 9. Divide by the largest number possible, namely, 9, to save extra steps.

$$\frac{27}{54} = \frac{9}{18} = \frac{1}{2}$$

Many drug calculations involve large fractions with several zeros in the numerator and the denominator. Reducing the fraction by dividing the numerator and denominator by 10, 100, or 1000 is termed *canceling zeros.*

Example 1.9: Reduce 200/400 to lowest terms.

Solution: The numerator and denominator are divisible by both 10 and 100.

$$\frac{200}{400}$$

Dividing by 10 yields:

$$\frac{200}{400} = \frac{20}{40} \text{ or } \frac{20\cancel{0}}{40\cancel{0}} = \frac{20}{40}$$

Dividing by 10 again yields:

$$\frac{20}{40} = \frac{2}{4} \text{ or } \frac{2\cancel{0}}{4\cancel{0}} = \frac{2}{4} = \frac{1}{2}$$

Note: If a zero is canceled in both the numerator and denominator, it is equivalent to dividing by 10.

▶ **SELF-TEST**

Reduce the following fractions to lowest terms.

1. $\dfrac{10}{15} =$ 2. $\dfrac{16}{24} =$

3. $\dfrac{4}{8} =$ 4. $\dfrac{10}{25} =$

Reduce the following fractions to lowest terms by first canceling zeros.

5. $\dfrac{250}{1000} =$ 6. $\dfrac{100}{300} =$

7. $\dfrac{500}{1000} =$ 8. $\dfrac{370}{630} =$

For answers to the self-test, see page 27.

Comparing Size (Magnitude) of Fractions

Some drugs are ordered in fractional quantities and dispensed from the pharmacy in solutions with a different fractional strength. It is very important that the nurse understands which fraction represents the greater amount of medication.

 When two fractions have *like numerators,* the fraction with the *smaller* denominator represents the *larger* fraction.   ◀ RULE

Always reduce fractions to lowest terms before comparing their magnitude. Applying the above rule to the two fractions, 1/32 and 1/64, one concludes that 1/64 represents the smaller fraction.

Example 1.10: Which fraction is larger: 1/6 or 1/3?

Solution: 1/3 is larger because the denominator is smaller, and 1/3 represents a greater part of the whole number 1.

Example 1.11: Which fraction is larger: 2/10 or 1/4?

Solution: Reduce 2/10 to lowest terms:

$$\frac{2}{10} = \frac{1}{5}$$

Next, compare 1/5 and 1/4. Since the numerators are equal, compare the magnitude of the denominators. 1/4 is larger because 4 is the smaller denominator.

RULE ▶ If two fractions have *like denominators*, the fraction with the *larger* numerator is the *larger* fraction.

Example 1.12: Which fraction is larger: 3/8 or 5/8?

Solution: 5/8 is larger. Since the denominators are equal, compare the magnitude of the numerators.

Example 1.13: Which fraction is larger: 1/2 or 4/8?

Solution: Reduce 4/8 to lowest terms:

$$\frac{4}{8} = \frac{1}{2}$$

Next, compare 1/2 and 1/2. The two fractions are equal!

RULE ▶ Fractions with *unlike* numerators and *unlike* denominators must be changed to fractions with *like* denominators before determining their magnitude.

Fractions with unlike denominators are converted to fractions with like denominators by finding the *common denominator* of both fractions. The common denominator is a number evenly divisible by the denominators of both fractions. For example, if one fraction has a denominator of 5 and a second fraction has a denominator of 3, the common denominator is 15. This is true because 15 is evenly divisible by both 5 and 3.

Example 1.14: Change 1/5 and 2/3 to like denominators and determine which fraction is larger.

Solution:

Step 1: Determine a common denominator for the two fractions.

   15 is the common denominator, since it is evenly divisible by both 3 and 5.

Step 2: Divide the denominator of each fraction into the common denominator. Then multiply the quotient by the numerator of each fraction.

$\dfrac{1}{5} = \dfrac{3}{15}$ Since $15 \div 5 = 3$, and $3 \times 1 = 3$. The 3 is the numerator of the new fraction.

Also:

$\dfrac{2}{3} = \dfrac{10}{15}$ Since $15 \div 3 = 5$, and $5 \times 2 = 10$. The 10 is the numerator of the new fraction.

Step 3: Determine the magnitude of the fractions. Which is larger: 3/15 or 10/15?

10/15 is larger. Therefore, 2/3 is the larger fraction.

▶ SELF-TEST

Determine the larger fraction in the pair of numbers.

1. $\dfrac{3}{8}, \dfrac{1}{6}$ 2. $\dfrac{2}{5}, \dfrac{1}{4}$

3. $\dfrac{3}{15}, \dfrac{2}{5}$ 4. $\dfrac{1}{4}, \dfrac{1}{6}$

Place the following fractions in order from lowest to highest value.

5. $\dfrac{1}{2}, \dfrac{1}{8}, \dfrac{1}{5}$ 6. $\dfrac{3}{7}, \dfrac{4}{7}, \dfrac{2}{5}$

7. $\dfrac{3}{5}, \dfrac{8}{5}, \dfrac{1}{5}$ 8. $\dfrac{1}{16}, \dfrac{1}{32}, \dfrac{1}{64}$

For answers to the self-test, see page 27.

Addition and Subtraction of Fractions

 To add or subtract fractions with like denominators, the denominator remains the same and the numerators are either added or subtracted.   ◀ RULE

Example 1.15:   *Example 1.16:*   *Example 1.17:*

$\dfrac{1}{9} + \dfrac{7}{9} = \dfrac{8}{9}$ $\dfrac{5}{11} + \dfrac{2}{11} = \dfrac{7}{11}$ $\dfrac{2}{8} + \dfrac{3}{8} = \dfrac{5}{8}$

Example 1.18:   *Example 1.19:*   *Example 1.20:*

$\dfrac{9}{13} - \dfrac{4}{13} = \dfrac{5}{13}$ $\dfrac{4}{7} - \dfrac{3}{7} = \dfrac{1}{7}$ $\dfrac{15}{22} - \dfrac{6}{22} = \dfrac{9}{22}$

 To add or subtract fractions with unlike denominators, find the least common denominator (L.C.D.) by finding the smallest number divisible by both denominators.   ◀ RULE

Example 1.21:

$\dfrac{2}{3} + \dfrac{1}{5}$ The smallest number divisible by both the 3 and the 5 is the number 15, the L.C.D.

Solution:

$\dfrac{2}{3} = \dfrac{10}{15}$ Divide each denominator into the number 15. Then multiply the quotient by the numerator.

$+\dfrac{1}{5} = \dfrac{3}{15}$

$\dfrac{13}{15}$

Answer: $\dfrac{13}{15}$

Example 1.22:

$\dfrac{2}{3} - \dfrac{1}{7}$ The smallest number divisible by both the 3 and the 7 is the number 21, the L.C.D.

Solution:

$\dfrac{2}{3} = \dfrac{14}{21}$ Divide each denominator into the number 21. Then multiply the quotient by the numerator.

$-\dfrac{1}{7} = \dfrac{3}{21}$

$\dfrac{11}{21}$

Answer: $\dfrac{11}{21}$

► SELF-TEST

Express your answer in lowest terms.

1. $\dfrac{3}{8} + \dfrac{1}{8} =$ 　　2. $\dfrac{2}{3} + \dfrac{1}{6} =$ 　　3. $\dfrac{3}{11} - \dfrac{1}{11} =$

4. $\dfrac{2}{3} - \dfrac{5}{12} =$ 　　4. $\dfrac{2}{7} + \dfrac{2}{3} =$ 　　6. $\dfrac{1}{2} - \dfrac{2}{9} =$

For answers to the self-test, see page 27.

Multiplication and Division of Fractions

 Multiplication of fractions is carried out by multiplying the numerators and then multiplying the denominators.

◀ RULE

$$\frac{4}{1} \times \frac{1}{4} = \frac{4}{4} = 1$$

Example 1.23:

$$\frac{1}{4} \times \frac{1}{2} \times \frac{3}{6} = \frac{3}{48}$$

Example 1.24:

$$\frac{1}{3} \times 4 \times \frac{2}{3} = \frac{8}{9}$$

Example 1.25:

$$\frac{1}{2} \times \frac{3}{5} \times \frac{7}{8} \times 3 = \frac{63}{80}$$

 Any numerator may be divided by any denominator, and any denominator may be divided by any numerator.

◀ RULE

Example 1.26:

$$\frac{2}{5} \times \frac{1}{6} \times \frac{10}{9} =$$ Divide 2 and 6 by 2, and 5 and 10 by 5. The resulting fractions are as follows:

$$\frac{1}{1} \times \frac{1}{3} \times \frac{2}{9} = \frac{2}{27}$$

Example 1.27:

$$\frac{30}{1} \times \frac{1}{60} \times \frac{250}{1000} =$$ First cancel the correct number of zeros to reduce the fractions. The resulting fractions are as follows:

$$\frac{3}{1} \times \frac{1}{6} \times \frac{25}{100} =$$ Divide 25 and 100 by 25, and 3 and 6 by 3. The resulting fractions are as follows:

$$\frac{1}{1} \times \frac{1}{2} \times \frac{1}{4} = \frac{1}{8}$$

 Division of fractions is accomplished by inverting the second fraction, then following the rules of multiplying fractions.

◀ RULE

Example 1.28:

$$\frac{1}{8} \div \frac{1}{3} = \quad \text{Invert the second fraction, then multiply.}$$

$$\frac{1}{8} \times \frac{3}{1} = \frac{3}{8}$$

Example 1.29:

$$\frac{4}{15} \div \frac{2}{3} = \frac{4}{15} \times \frac{3}{2} = \quad$$ Divide 4 and 2 by 2, and 3 and 15 by 5. The resulting fractions are as follows:

$$\frac{2}{5} \times \frac{1}{1} = \frac{2}{5}$$

Example 1.30:

$$\frac{2}{5} \div 3 = \frac{2}{5} \times \frac{1}{3} = \frac{2}{15}$$

► **SELF-TEST**

Express your answers in lowest terms.

1. $\dfrac{5}{8} \times \dfrac{7}{8} =$ 2. $\dfrac{2}{4} \times \dfrac{6}{9} =$ 3. $\dfrac{5}{6} \times 3 =$

4. $\dfrac{1}{12} \div \dfrac{1}{3} =$ 5. $\dfrac{2}{15} \div \dfrac{2}{3} =$ 6. $\dfrac{5}{6} \div 10 =$

For answers to the self-test, see page 27.

▲ MIXED NUMBERS AND IMPROPER FRACTIONS

A mixed number has a whole number and a fraction. An improper fraction is a fraction with a numerator that is larger than the denominator. Improper fractions can be converted to mixed numbers, and mixed numbers can be converted to improper fractions.

RULE ► When changing an improper fraction to a mixed number, divide the numerator by the denominator. The quotient becomes the whole number and the remainder is the numerator of the new fraction.

Example 1.31:   *Example 1.32:*

$$\frac{13}{12} = 1\frac{1}{12} \qquad\qquad \frac{17}{3} = 5\frac{2}{3}$$

When changing a mixed number to an improper fraction, multiply the whole number by the denominator, then add to that product the numerator. The resulting number is the numerator of the improper fraction.

◀ RULE

Example 1.33:

$$2\frac{1}{4} = \frac{9}{4}$$

Example 1.34:

$$6\frac{2}{5} = \frac{32}{5}$$

 When adding or subtracting mixed numbers, it is always necessary to have a common denominator.

◀ RULE

Example 1.35:

$$2\frac{1}{6} = 2\frac{1}{6}$$
$$+ 1\frac{1}{2} = 1\frac{3}{6}$$
$$\overline{3\frac{4}{6} = 3\frac{2}{3}}$$

Answer: $3\frac{2}{3}$

Example 1.36:

$$6\frac{1}{3} = 6\frac{4}{12}$$
$$- 2\frac{1}{4} = 2\frac{3}{12}$$
$$\overline{4\frac{1}{12}}$$

Answer: $4\frac{1}{12}$

 Mixed numbers are multiplied or divided by first converting to improper fractions.

◀ RULE

Example 1.37:

$$2\frac{1}{4} \times 3\frac{1}{2} = \frac{9}{4} \times \frac{7}{2} = \frac{63}{8} = 7\frac{7}{8}$$

Example 1.38:

$$3\frac{2}{5} \div 2\frac{6}{7} = \frac{17}{5} \div \frac{20}{7}, \text{ then}$$

$$\frac{17}{5} \times \frac{7}{20} = \frac{119}{100} = 1\frac{19}{100}$$

▶ **SELF-TEST**

Express your answers as whole or mixed numbers in lowest terms.

1. $6\frac{1}{2} + 2\frac{1}{2} =$ 2. $8\frac{2}{3} - 4\frac{1}{2} =$

3. $2\frac{1}{2} \times 3\frac{1}{2} =$ 4. $4\frac{3}{4} \div 2\frac{1}{3} =$

For answers to the self-test, see page 27.

▲ DECIMALS

Defining Decimal Places

- Numbers are defined by their position in reference to the decimal place.

0. 2 3 5 6 7 4
.   .   .   .   .   .   millionths
.   .   .   .   .   hundred thousandths
.   .   .   .   ten thousandths
.   .   .   thousandths
.   .   hundredths
.   tenths

- Whole numbers are similarly defined in reference to the decimal place.

2 6 8 7 2
.   .   .   .   .   ones
.   .   .   .   tens
.   .   .   hundreds
.   .   thousands
.   ten thousands

Rounding Decimals

If the last digit in a number is 5, 6, 7, 8, or 9 increase the digit to the left of it by one. If the last digit is 1, 2, 3, 4 then drop the last digit. With decimal numbers it is often necessary to round to the nearest tenth, hundredth, or thousandth.

Example 1.39: Round 1.346 to the nearest tenth (one decimal place).
The 4 in the hundredth place is dropped along with any numbers to the right of it. The rounded number is 1.3.

Example 1.40: Round 1.346 to the nearest hundredth (two decimal places).
Since there is a 6 in the thousandth place, the 4 in the hundredth place is increased by 5. The rounded number is 1.35.

Example 1.41: Round 0.2893456 to the nearest thousandth (three decimal places).
Since there is a 3 in the fourth decimal place, the 3 is dropped along with any numbers to the right of it. The rounded number is 0.289.

▶ SELF-TEST

Round to the nearest tenth.

1. 0.07 =   2. 0.24 =   3. 3.46 =

Round to the nearest hundredth.

4. 0.357 =   5. 0.591 =   6. 5.555 =

For answers to the self-test, see page 27.

Comparing Size (Magnitude) of Decimals

To compare two decimals, add enough zeros to the right of the last digit in order that the numbers have the same number of decimal places.

Example 1.42: Place in order from lowest to highest value.

0.25, 0.2, 0.21

Solution: Add the appropriate number of zeros.

0.25, 0.20, 0.21

Answer: 0.20, 0.21, 0.25

Example 1.43: Place in order from lowest to highest.

0.01, 0.002, 0.12

Solution: Add the appropriate number of zeros.

0.010, 0.002, 0.120

Answer: 0.002, 0.010, 0.120

▶ SELF-TEST

Rank in order of size from lowest to highest.

1. 0.5, 0.05, 0.521
2. 0.3, 0.06, 0.81
3. 1.01, 1.11, 1.101
4. 1.9, 1.91, 9.19

For answers to the self-test, see page 28.

Addition and Subtraction of Decimals

 When adding or subtracting decimals, place the numbers in a column with the decimal points aligned.

◀ RULE

Example 1.44: Add 1.256 + 0.12 + 12.3

Solution:

1.256	Zeros may be added	1.256
0.12	to the right of the last	0.120
+ 12.3	digit if desired.	+ 12.300
13.676		13.676

► **SELF-TEST**

Express to the nearest tenth.

1. $3.2 + 0.43 =$ 2. $6.5 - 0.4 =$

Express to the nearest hundredth.

3. $12.03 + 102.113 =$ 4. $15.25 - 1.891 =$

For answers to the self-test, see page 28.

Multiplication and Division of Decimals

RULE ► When multiplying decimal numbers, the product contains as many decimal places as the sum of the decimal places in the numbers being multiplied.

Example 1.45: Multiply 22.3×4.12

Solution: The number 22.3 has one decimal place. The number 4.12 has two decimal places. The final answer has three decimal places.

```
      22.3
  ×   4.12
      446
     223
     892
   91876   Put the decimal three places to the left to give: 91.876
```

Answer: $22.3 \times 4.12 = 91.876$

Example 1.46: Divide $3.5 \div 2.5 = 2.5\overline{)3.5} =$

Solution:

```
      1.4
 25.)35.0
      25
      100
      100
```

When the divisor is a decimal number, it must be converted to a whole number by moving the decimal place the same number of places in the divisor and the dividend.

Answer: $3.5 \div 2.5 = 1.4$

▶ SELF-TEST

Express to the nearest tenth.

1. $12 \times 3.2 =$ 2. $0.7 \div 0.3 =$

Express to the nearest hundredth.

3. $1.2 \times 5.22 =$ 4. $3.6 \div 4.2 =$

For answers to the self-test, see page 28.

Changing Fractions to Decimals

 To change a fraction to a decimal, the numerator is divided by the denominator.

◀ RULE

Example 1.47:   *Example 1.48:*

$$\frac{4}{5} = \begin{array}{r} 0.8 \\ 5)\overline{4.0} \\ \underline{4\,0} \end{array}$$

$$\frac{150}{200} = \begin{array}{r} 0.75 \\ 200)\overline{150.00} \\ \underline{140\,0} \\ 100\,0 \\ \underline{100\,0} \end{array}$$

▶ SELF-TEST

Express to the nearest tenth.

1. $\dfrac{4}{9}$ 2. $\dfrac{150}{200}$

3. $\dfrac{1}{5}$ 4. $\dfrac{60}{40}$

For answers to the self-test, see page 28.

Multiplication and Division by 10, 100, and 1000

Notice that

10 has one zero.
100 has two zeros.
1000 has three zeros.

RULE ▶ To *multiply* by 10, 100, or 1000, count the number of zeros and move the decimal point that number of places to the *right*.

Example 1.49:

$2.56 \times 10 =$

Solution: 10 has one zero. Therefore move the decimal *one* place to the *right* to increase its value.

Answer: $2.56 \times 10 = 25.6$

Example 1.50:

$36.10 \times 1000 =$

Solution: 1000 has 3 zeros. Move the decimal point *three* places to the *right* to increase its value.

Answer: $36.10 \times 1000 = 36,100$

RULE ▶ To *divide* by 10, 100, or 1000, count the number of zeros and move the decimal point that number of places to the *left*.

Example 1.51:

$0.235 \div 10 =$

Solution: 10 has one zero. Move the decimal point *one* place to the *left* to decrease its value.

Answer: $0.235 \div 10 = 0.0235$

Example 1.52:

$36.15 \div 100 =$

Solution: 100 has two zeros. Move the decimal point *two* places to the *left* to decrease its value.

Answer: $36.15 \div 100 = 0.3615$

▶ SELF-TEST

Complete the following multiplication and division problems.

1. $23 \times 10 =$ 　　2. $13.2 \times 100 =$ 　　3. $0.456 \times 1000 =$
4. $15 \div 10 =$ 　　5. $0.67 \div 100 =$ 　　6. $350 \div 100 =$

For answers to the self-test, see page 28.

SIMPLIFYING COMPLEX FRACTIONS

In complex fractions, the numerator, the denominator, or both contain a fraction. The complex fraction is converted into a simple fraction, a mixed number, a decimal number, or a whole number when it is simplified.

To simplify a complex fraction, invert the denominator and multiply the numerator by the denominator.	◄ RULE

Example 1.53:

$$\frac{2}{\frac{1}{2}} = 2 \div \frac{1}{2} = 2 \times \frac{2}{1} = 4$$

Example 1.54:

$$\frac{\frac{1}{100}}{\frac{1}{4}} = \frac{1}{100} \div \frac{1}{4} = \frac{1}{100} \times \frac{4}{1} = \frac{4}{100} = \frac{1}{25}$$

► SELF-TEST

Simplify the following complex fractions and express your answer in lowest terms.

1. $\dfrac{\frac{1}{5}}{\frac{2}{3}} =$ 　　　2. $\dfrac{4}{\frac{2}{3}} =$ 　　　3. $\dfrac{\frac{1}{50}}{\frac{1}{5}} =$

For answers to the self-test, see page 28.

▲ PERCENT

Percent is used in nursing to express the concentration of a given solution. For example, 3% saline solution means that there are three parts of saline to 100 parts of water. Like a fraction, a percent represents a part of a whole.

Changing Decimals to Percents

To change a decimal to a percent, multiply by 100, moving the decimal point two places to the *right*.	◄ RULE

Example 1.55:

$0.15 \times 100 = 15\%$

Example 1.56:

$0.09 \times 100 = 9\%$

▶ **SELF-TEST**

Express the following decimals as percents.

1. 0.32   2. 0.06   3. 0.001
4. 0.6   5. 0.51   6. 0.0025

For answers to the self-test, see page 28.

Changing Fractions to Percents

RULE ▶ To change a fraction to a percent, change the fraction to a decimal and then change the decimal to a percent.

Example 1.57: Change 1/4 to a percent.

Solution:

1/4 = 0.25, then 0.25 × 100 = 25%

Answer: 1/4 = 25%

Example 1.58: Change 2/5 to a percent.

Solution:

2/5 = 0.4, then 0.4 × 100 = 40%

Answer: 2/5 = 40%

▶ **SELF-TEST**

Change the following fractions to percents.

1. $\dfrac{4}{5}$ 2. $\dfrac{1}{3}$ 3. $\dfrac{9}{10}$

4. $\dfrac{3}{4}$ 5. $\dfrac{1}{8}$ 6. $\dfrac{25}{75}$

For answers to the self-test, see page 28.

Changing a Percent to a Decimal

RULE ▶ Change a percent to a decimal by dividing by 100, or moving the decimal point to the *left* two places, and dropping the percent sign.

Example 1.59: Change 23% to a decimal.

Solution:

23% = 23/100 = 0.23

Answer: 23% = 0.23

Alternate Solution: 23% has a decimal understood to the right of the number. Move this decimal to the left two places and drop the percent sign.

Answer: 23% = 0.23

Example 1.60: Change 0.9% to a decimal.

Solution:

0.9% = 0.9/100 = 0.009

Answer: 0.9% = 0.009

Alternate Solution: Move the decimal to the left two places and drop the percent sign.

Answer: 0.9% = 0.009

▶ **SELF-TEST**

Change the following percents to decimals.

1. 18%   2. 9.3%   3. 4.13%
4. 62%   5. 25.4%   6. 0.45%

For answers to the self-test, see page 28.

Multiplying by a Percent

 To multiply by a percent, change the percent to a decimal, and then multiply by the given number.

◀ RULE

Example 1.61: What is 26% of 52?

Solution:

    Step 1:   26% = 26/100 = 0.26
    Step 2:   0.26 × 52 = 13.52

Answer: 26% of 52 = 13.52

Example 1.62: What is 2.65% of 90?

Solution:

    Step 1:   2.65% = 2.65/100 = 0.0265
    Step 2:   0.0265 × 90 = 2.385

Answer: 2.65% of 90 = 2.385

Finding the Percent One Number is of Another

The percent one number is of another is equal to the fractional part of the given number.

RULE ►

> The percent one number is of another is determined by expressing the numbers as a fraction. The fraction is converted to a decimal and the resulting decimal is then converted to a percent.

Example 1.63: What percent of 20 is 5?

Solution:

Step 1: $\dfrac{5}{20} = 0.25$

Step 2: $0.25 \times 100 = 25\%$

Answer: 5 is 25% of 20

Example 1.64: What percent of 75 is 30?

Solution:

Step 1: $\dfrac{30}{75} = 0.40$

Step 2: $0.40 \times 100 = 40\%$

Answer: 30 is 40% of 75

▲ POST-TEST OF ARITHMETIC SKILLS

Roman Numerals

1. Write the following as Arabic numbers.

    A. vii   B. ix   C. xx

2. Write the Roman numeral that corresponds to each number.

    A. 5   B. 2   C. 14

Reducing Fractions

3. Reduce the following fractions to lowest terms.

    A. $\dfrac{3}{9}$ B. $\dfrac{7}{28}$ C. $\dfrac{10}{15}$

    D. $\dfrac{150}{300}$ E. $\dfrac{120}{360}$ F. $\dfrac{2}{10}$

Comparing the Magnitude of Fractions

4. Determine the larger fraction in the pair of numbers.

    A. $\dfrac{1}{8}, \dfrac{1}{9}$ B. $\dfrac{2}{5}, \dfrac{1}{10}$ C. $\dfrac{3}{6}, \dfrac{4}{7}$

5. Place the following fractions in order from lowest to highest.

    A. $\dfrac{1}{6}, \dfrac{1}{9}, \dfrac{1}{3}$ B. $\dfrac{2}{3}, \dfrac{5}{9}, \dfrac{3}{5}$ C. $\dfrac{2}{4}, \dfrac{1}{5}, \dfrac{3}{10}$

Addition and Subtraction of Fractions

6. Add or subtract the following fractions. Express your answer in lowest terms.

    A. $\dfrac{3}{4} - \dfrac{1}{5} =$ B. $\dfrac{4}{5} - \dfrac{1}{5} =$ C. $\dfrac{3}{8} - \dfrac{1}{4} =$

    D. $\dfrac{2}{3} + \dfrac{1}{6} =$ E. $\dfrac{5}{16} + \dfrac{1}{8} + \dfrac{1}{2} =$ F. $\dfrac{4}{7} + \dfrac{1}{2} =$

Multiplication and Division of Fractions

7. Multiply or divide the following fractions. Express your answer in lowest terms.

    A. $\dfrac{1}{3} \times \dfrac{1}{2} =$ B. $\dfrac{4}{5} \times \dfrac{10}{14} =$ C. $\dfrac{2}{7} \times 4 \times \dfrac{1}{2} =$

    D. $\dfrac{1}{9} \div \dfrac{3}{18} =$ E. $\dfrac{5}{6} \div \dfrac{2}{3} =$ F. $\dfrac{2}{7} \div \dfrac{4}{9} =$

Mixed Numbers and Improper Fractions

8. Express your answers as whole or mixed numbers in lowest terms.

    A. $2\dfrac{2}{3} + \dfrac{1}{3} =$ B. $3\dfrac{1}{7} - 2 =$ C. $\dfrac{13}{3} + \dfrac{7}{3} =$

    D. $\dfrac{2}{5} \div 2\dfrac{1}{2} =$ E. $4\dfrac{1}{2} \times \dfrac{2}{5} =$ F. $6 \times 1\dfrac{4}{5} =$

Comparing the Magnitude of Decimals

9. Place in order from lowest to highest value.
   A. 0.2, 0.27, 0.17
   B. 0.02, 0.21, 0.5
   C. 0.4, 0.45, 0.6
   D. 1.010, 10.100, 0.100
   E. 3.3, 3.03, 0.303
   F. 0.099, 0.909, 0.9

Addition, Subtraction, Multiplication, and Division of Decimals

10. Express all answers to the nearest tenth.
    A. $6.23 + 0.51 =$
    B. $4.6 - 2.51 =$
    C. $12 \times 2.5 =$
    D. $1.25 \times 0.3 =$
    E. $15 \div 1.3 =$
    F. $2.75 \div 3 =$

Changing Fractions to Decimals

11. Change the following fractions to decimals and express the answer to the nearest hundredth.

    A. $\dfrac{2}{5} =$
    B. $\dfrac{3}{7} =$
    C. $\dfrac{3}{4} =$

    D. $\dfrac{10}{12} =$
    E. $\dfrac{20}{25} =$
    F. $\dfrac{4}{8} =$

Multiplication and Division by 10, 100, and 1000

12. Multiply or divide the following by moving the decimal point the appropriate number of places.
    A. $1.3 \times 10 =$
    B. $14 \times 100 =$
    C. $0.31 \times 10 =$

    D. $125 \div 1000 =$
    E. $\dfrac{750}{1000} =$
    F. $\dfrac{50}{10} =$

Simplifying Complex Fractions

13. Simplify the following complex fractions and express your answer in lowest terms.

    A. $\dfrac{\frac{1}{4}}{\frac{1}{8}} =$
    B. $\dfrac{\frac{1}{200}}{\frac{1}{150}} =$
    C. $\dfrac{\frac{1}{3}}{\frac{1}{4}} =$

    D. $\dfrac{75}{\frac{1}{0.5}} =$
    E. $\dfrac{\frac{0.5}{3}}{\frac{1}{3}} =$
    F. $\dfrac{\frac{2}{5}}{\frac{1}{5}} =$

Changing Decimals and Fractions to Percents

14. Change the following to percents.
    A. 0.23
    B. 0.05
    C. 0.33

    D. $\dfrac{1}{6}$
    E. $\dfrac{1}{3}$
    F. $\dfrac{2}{5}$

Calculations with Percent

15. Change the following percents to decimals.

    A. 0.45%   B. 3.1%   C. 20%

16. Multiply the following numbers by the given percent.

    A. What is 9% of 18?

    B. What is 40% of 14.2?

    C. What is 3.5% of 14?

17. Find the percent one number is of another.

    A. What percent of 15 is 5?

    B. What percent of 100 is 13?

    C. What percent of 40 is 10?

For answers to the post-test, see page 29.

The prerequisite test that you have completed is divided into several sections. If you have any incorrect answers, review that section of Chapter 1 and then complete the corresponding parts of the post-test on page 23.

Roman Numerals

1. A. 12	B. 4	C. 25
2. A. vi	B. xiii	C. xix

Reducing Fractions

3. A. $\frac{1}{3}$ B. $\frac{1}{4}$ C. $\frac{2}{3}$

   D. $\frac{1}{2}$ E. $\frac{1}{3}$ F. $\frac{1}{2}$

Comparing the Magnitude of Fractions

4. A. $\frac{1}{16}$ B. $\frac{2}{3}$ C. $\frac{2}{4}$

5. A. $\frac{1}{6}, \frac{1}{4}, \frac{1}{3}$ B. $\frac{3}{7}, \frac{2}{3}, \frac{5}{6}$ C. $\frac{2}{10}, \frac{1}{4}, \frac{2}{3}$

Addition and Subtraction of Fractions

6. A. $\frac{1}{2}$ B. $\frac{1}{4}$ C. $\frac{1}{14}$

   D. $1\frac{1}{10}$ E. 1   F. $\frac{25}{42}$

ANSWERS to Prerequisite Test of Arithmetic Skills

Multiplication and Division of Fractions

7. A. $\dfrac{1}{6}$

    B. $\dfrac{5}{12}$

    C. $\dfrac{1}{5}$

    D. 2

    E. $1\dfrac{2}{3}$

    F. 2

Mixed Numbers and Improper Fractions

8. A. 2

    B. $4\dfrac{35}{36}$

    C. $2\dfrac{1}{6}$

    D. $\dfrac{3}{4}$

    E. $\dfrac{5}{6}$

    F. $\dfrac{5}{6}$

Comparing the Magnitude of Decimals

9. A. 0.3, 0.32, 0.37   B. 0.02, 0.1, 0.4   C. 0.35, 0.6, 0.75

    D. 0.009, 0.900, 0.909   E. 0.021, 0.12, 0.21   F. 0.155, 0.515, 0.551

Addition, Subtraction, Multiplication, and Division of Decimals

10. A. 4.6   B. 2.3   C. 32.2

    D. 0.5   E. 2.0   F. 3.0

Changing Fractions to Decimals

11. A. 0.4   B. 0.3   C. 0.7

    D. 0.9   E. 0.8   F. 0.6

Multiplication and Division by 10, 100, and 1000

12. A. 120   B. 2500   C. 3.2

    D. 1.50   E. 0.250   F. 1.25

Simplifying Complex Fractions

13. A. 3   B. 1.3   C. 0.1

    D. 1500   E. 1   F. 4

Changing Decimals and Fractions to Percents

14. A. 17%   B. 9%   C. 66%

    D. 50%   E. 25%   F. 80%

Calculations with Percent

15. A. 0.0085   B. 0.023   C. 0.25

16. A. 4.32   B. 0.99   C. 0.384

17. A. 20%   B. 9%   C. 20%

Roman Numerals

1. 13   2. 7   3. 9   4. 24
5. 15   6. ii   7. xi   8. xvi
9. viii   10. xxv

Common Fractions

Reducing Fractions

1. $\dfrac{2}{3}$ 2. $\dfrac{2}{3}$ 3. $\dfrac{1}{2}$ 4. $\dfrac{2}{5}$

5. $\dfrac{1}{4}$ 6. $\dfrac{1}{3}$ 7. $\dfrac{1}{2}$ 8. $\dfrac{37}{63}$

Comparing Size (Magnitude) of Fractions

1. $\dfrac{3}{8}$ 2. $\dfrac{2}{5}$ 3. $\dfrac{2}{5}$

4. $\dfrac{1}{4}$ 5. $\dfrac{1}{8}, \dfrac{1}{5}, \dfrac{1}{2}$ 6. $\dfrac{2}{5}, \dfrac{3}{7}, \dfrac{4}{7}$

7. $\dfrac{1}{5}, \dfrac{3}{5}, \dfrac{8}{5}$ 8. $\dfrac{1}{64}, \dfrac{1}{32}, \dfrac{1}{16}$

Addition and Subtraction of Fractions

1. $\dfrac{1}{2}$ 2. $\dfrac{5}{6}$ 3. $\dfrac{2}{11}$

4. $\dfrac{1}{4}$ 5. $\dfrac{20}{21}$ 6. $\dfrac{5}{18}$

Multiplication and Division of Fractions

1. $\dfrac{35}{64}$ 2. $\dfrac{1}{3}$ 3. $2\dfrac{1}{2}$

4. $\dfrac{1}{4}$ 5. $\dfrac{1}{5}$ 6. $\dfrac{1}{12}$

Mixed Numbers and Improper Fractions

1. 9   2. $4\dfrac{1}{6}$ 3. $8\dfrac{3}{4}$ 4. $2\dfrac{1}{28}$

Decimals

Rounding Decimals

1. 0.1   2. 0.2   3. 3.5
4. 0.36   5. 0.59   6. 5.56

Comparing Size (Magnitude) of Decimals
1. 0.05, 0.5, 0.521   2. 0.06, 0.3, 0.81
3. 1.01, 1.101, 1.11   4. 1.9, 1.91, 9.19

Addition and Subtraction of Decimals
1. 3.6   2. 6.1   3. 114.14   4. 13.36

Multiplication and Division of Decimals
1. 38.4   2. 2.3   3. 6.26   4. 0.86

Changing Fractions to Decimals
1. 0.4   2. 0.8   3. 0.2   4. 1.5

Multiplication and Division by 10, 100, and 1000
1. 230   2. 1320   3. 456
4. 1.5   5. 0.0067   6. 3.5

Simplifying Complex Fractions

1. $\dfrac{3}{10}$ 2. 6   3. $\dfrac{1}{10}$

Percent

Changing Decimals to Percents
1. 32%   2. 6%   3. 0.1%
4. 60%   5. 51%   6. 0.25%

Changing Fractions to Percents
1. 80%   2. 33.3%   3. 90%
4. 75%   5. 12.5%   6. 33.3%

Changing a Percent to a Decimal
1. 0.18   2. 0.093   3. 0.0413
4. 0.62   6. 0.254   6. 0.0045

Multiplying by a Percent
1. 4.2   2. 0.45   3. 0.625
4. 0.14   5. 4.575   6. 0.2

Finding the Percent One Number Is of Another
1. 20%   2. 16.7%   3. 33.3%   4. 50%

Roman Numerals

1. A. 7   B. 9   C. 20
2. A. v   B. ii   C. xiv

Reducing Fractions

3. A. $\frac{1}{3}$ B. $\frac{1}{4}$ C. $\frac{2}{3}$

    D. $\frac{1}{2}$ E. $\frac{1}{3}$ F. $\frac{1}{5}$

Comparing the Magnitude of Fractions

4. A. $\frac{1}{8}$ B. $\frac{2}{5}$ C. $\frac{4}{7}$

5. A. $\frac{1}{9}, \frac{1}{6}, \frac{1}{3}$ B. $\frac{5}{9}, \frac{3}{5}, \frac{2}{3}$ C. $\frac{1}{5}, \frac{3}{10}, \frac{2}{4}$

Addition and Subtraction of Fractions

6. A. $\frac{11}{20}$ B. $\frac{3}{5}$ C. $\frac{1}{8}$

    D. $\frac{5}{6}$ E. $\frac{15}{16}$ F. $1\frac{1}{14}$

Multiplication and Division of Fractions

7. A. $\frac{1}{6}$ B. $\frac{4}{7}$ C. $\frac{4}{7}$

    D. $\frac{2}{3}$ E. $1\frac{1}{4}$ F. $\frac{9}{14}$

Mixed Numbers and Improper Fractions

8. A. 3   B. $1\frac{1}{7}$ C. $6\frac{2}{3}$

    D. $\frac{4}{25}$ E. $1\frac{4}{5}$ F. $10\frac{4}{5}$

Comparing the Magnitude of Decimals

9. A. 0.17, 0.2, 0.27   B. 0.02, 0.21, 0.5   C. 0.4, 0.45, 0.6
    D. 0.100, 1.010, 10.100   E. 0.303, 3.03, 3.3   F. 0.099, 0.9, 0.909

Addition, Subtraction, Multiplication, and Division of Decimals

10. A. 6.7   B. 2.1   C. 30
    D. 0.4   E. 11.5   F. 0.9

Changing Fractions to Decimals

11. A. 0.40   B. 0.43   C. 0.75

     D. 0.83   E. 0.80   F. 0.50

Multiplication and Division by 10, 100, and 1000

12. A. 13   B. 1400   C. 3.1

     D. 0.125   E. 0.75   F. 5

Simplifying Complex Fractions

13. A. 2   B. $\dfrac{3}{4}$ C. $\dfrac{1}{12}$

     D. 37.5   E. 0.5   F. 2

Changing Decimals and Fractions to Percents

14. A. 23%   B. 5%   C. 33%

     D. 16.7%   E. 33.3%   F. 40%

Calculations with Percent

15. A. 0.0045   16. A. 1.62   17. A. 33.3%

     B. 0.031   B. 5.68   B. 13%

     C. 0.20   C. 0.49   C. 25%

The Dimensional Analysis Method of Problem Solving

2

Upon completion of Chapter 2, the student will be able to:

▶ Recall the definition of a conversion factor.

▶ State the two rules of problem solving by dimensional analysis.

▶ Apply the rules of problem solving by dimensional analysis to correctly calculate equivalent quantities of length and weight.

▲ INTRODUCTION TO DIMENSIONAL ANALYSIS

Dimensional analysis, also known as the factor-label method of problem solving, is a refinement of the well-known ratio and proportion method. It is widely used in science and is applicable to all dosage calculations based on direct proportions. Because of its universal application to drug dosage and intravenous fluid calculations, no other method of problem solving need be used. Therefore, the necessity to learn multiple formulas for solving different types of problems is eliminated.

Dimensional analysis provides a system of checks to determine whether or not a given problem has been set up correctly prior to calculating the answer. This method eliminates the most frequent types of calculation errors made.

Definitions

1. *Dimensional analysis* is defined as a problem-solving method that changes one unit of measurement to another by multiplying a particular unit of measurement by a conversion factor.

2. A *conversion factor* is a factor that produces a change in the form of a quantity or expression without changing its value.

Example: Since 1 foot is equal to 12 inches, the conversion factor can be expressed as: 1 foot = 12 inches. This conversion factor may also be expressed as: 1 foot per 12 inches or as 12 inches per 1 foot.

The conversion factor may be used in calculations in either of two possible fractional forms:

$$\frac{1 \text{ foot}}{12 \text{ inches}} \quad \text{or} \quad \frac{12 \text{ inches}}{1 \text{ foot}}$$

Multiplying the quantity *24 inches* by a conversion factor will result in a change in form but not a change in value.

$$24 \text{ inches} \times \frac{1 \text{ foot}}{12 \text{ inches}} = 2 \text{ feet}$$

The final expression, *2 feet,* is equal to the original value of *24 inches.* Multiplying by a conversion factor has resulted in a change of form from inches to feet but not in a change of value.

Additional examples of conversion factors are given below.

1. 2 pounds = ? ounces   Conversion factor: $\frac{16 \text{ oz}}{1 \text{ lb}}$

$$2 \text{ lb} \times \frac{16 \text{ oz}}{1 \text{ lb}} = 32 \text{ oz}$$

The conversion factor is *16 oz per 1 lb.* Multiplying *2 lb* by the conversion factor gives *32 oz,* which is equal to *2 lb.*

2. 2 yards = ? feet   Conversion factor: $\frac{3 \text{ ft}}{1 \text{ yd}}$

$$2 \text{ yd} \times \frac{3 \text{ ft}}{1 \text{ yd}} = 6 \text{ ft}$$

The conversion factor is *3 ft per 1 yd.* Multiplying *2 yd* by the conversion factor gives *6 ft,* which is equal to *2 yd.*

3. 3000 pounds = ? tons   Conversion factor: $\frac{1 \text{ ton}}{2000 \text{ lb}}$

$$3000 \text{ lb} \times \frac{1 \text{ ton}}{2000 \text{ lb}} = 1.5 \text{ tons}$$

The conversion factor is *1 ton per 2000 lb.* Multiplying *3000 lb* by the conversion factor gives *1.5 tons,* which is equal to *3000 lb.*

▲ PROBLEM SOLVING BY DIMENSIONAL ANALYSIS

The dimensional analysis method of problem solving is illustrated in the solution to the problem: How many feet are equal to 42 inches?

One side of an equation can be multiplied by a conversion factor without changing the value of the equation.

▶ Application of Rule 1

In the problem given above, the solution requires converting from inches to feet. This conversion requires the use of a known conversion factor that relates feet to inches. That conversion factor is: 1 foot = 12 inches. This conversion factor can be put into the problem in one of two possible forms:

1 foot = 12 inches gives $\dfrac{1\ \text{ft}}{12\ \text{in}}$ or $\dfrac{12\ \text{in}}{1\ \text{ft}}$

 The problem is correctly set up when all labels cancel from both the numerator and the denominator except the label that is desired in the answer.

▶ Application of Rule 2

1. In the problem given, the question asked is how many feet are equal to 42 inches?
2. Stated in an equation form, the problem is

   $x\ \text{ft} = 42\ \text{in}$

   The letter "x" stands for the unknown quantity, or for the number of feet that are equal to 42 inches.
3. The conversion factor, 1 foot = 12 inches, is put into the equation as a fraction. The form of the fraction used is that which will cancel the unwanted label (inches) and leave only the desired label (feet).

   $x\ \text{ft} = 42\ \text{in} \times \dfrac{1\ \text{ft}}{12\ \text{in}}$

   The equation can be read: x feet equals 42 inches when it is true that there is 1 foot per 12 inches.
4. Cancel labels that appear in both the numerator and denominator on the *same* side of the equal sign.

   $x\ \text{ft} = 42\ \text{in} \times \dfrac{1\ \text{ft}}{12\ \text{in}}$

   The label *inches* cancels from both the numerator and denominator, leaving only the label, feet, on each side of the equal sign. Since the label desired in the final answer is feet, and this is the *only* label left in the problem, the problem is *correctly* set up. The form of the equation that remains after the cancellation of like labels is

   $x\ \text{ft} = 42 \times \dfrac{1\ \text{ft}}{12}$

5. Complete the required mathematical operations.

$$x = \frac{42 \times 1 \text{ ft}}{12} = \frac{7 \times 1 \text{ ft}}{2} = 3.5 \text{ ft}$$

Therefore, 3.5 feet = 42 inches.

The method of problem solving by dimensional analysis illustrated above is used throughout this unit. This same method is applicable to all types of dosage calculations and is used throughout the entire book.

Calculations Requiring One Conversion Factor

Example 2.1 is similar to the problem worked above. This example requires using only one conversion factor and involves working with simple fractions.

Example 2.1: How many yards are equal to 39 feet?

Step 1: State the problem in equation form.

x yd = 39 ft

Step 2: Identify the conversion factor needed to convert from feet to yards: 1 yard = 3 feet.

1 yard = 3 feet gives $\dfrac{1 \text{ yd}}{3 \text{ ft}}$ or $\dfrac{3 \text{ ft}}{1 \text{ yd}}$

Step 3: Put into the equation the form of the conversion factor that will cancel the unwanted label (feet) and leave only the desired label (yards) on both sides of the equal sign.

x yd = 39 ft $\times \dfrac{1 \text{ yd}}{3 \text{ ft}}$

The equation can be read: x yards equal 39 feet when it is true that there is 1 yard per 3 feet.

Step 4: Cancel the labels that appear in both the numerator and the denominator on the same side of the equal sign.

x yd = 39 $\times \dfrac{1 \text{ yd}}{3}$

Step 5: Complete the required mathematical operations.

$$x \text{ yd} = \frac{39 \times 1 \text{ yd}}{3} = \frac{13 \times 1 \text{ yd}}{1} = 13 \text{ yd}$$

Therefore, 13 yards = 39 feet.

Calculations Requiring More Than One Conversion Factor

Example 2.2 requires working with more than one conversion factor. Once again it will be necessary to put into the equation the form of each conversion factor that will cancel the unwanted labels from the equation.

Example 2.2: How many inches are in 1 mile?

Step 1: State the problem in equation form.

x in = 1 mile

Step 2: Identify the conversion factors needed to convert from miles to inches. Three conversion factors are needed:

A. Convert from miles to yards

1 mile = 1760 yards gives $\dfrac{1 \text{ mile}}{1760 \text{ yd}}$ or $\dfrac{1760 \text{ yd}}{1 \text{ mile}}$

B. Convert from yards to feet.

1 yard = 3 feet gives $\dfrac{1 \text{ yd}}{3 \text{ ft}}$ or $\dfrac{3 \text{ ft}}{1 \text{ yd}}$

C. Convert from feet to inches.

1 foot = 12 inches gives $\dfrac{1 \text{ ft}}{12 \text{ in}}$ or $\dfrac{12 \text{ in}}{1 \text{ ft}}$

Step 3: Put into the equation the form of each conversion factor that will cancel the unwanted labels (miles, yards, and feet) and leave only the desired label (inches) on both sides of the equal sign.

$$x \text{ in} = 1 \text{ mile} \times \dfrac{1760 \text{ yd}}{1 \text{ mile}} \times \dfrac{3 \text{ ft}}{1 \text{ yd}} \times \dfrac{12 \text{ in}}{1 \text{ ft}}$$

The equation can be read: x inches equal 1 mile when it is true that there are 1760 yards per 1 mile, and when it is true that there are 3 feet per 1 yard, and when it is true that there are 12 inches per 1 foot.

Step 4: Cancel the labels that appear in both the numerator and the denominator on the same side of the equal sign.

$$x \text{ in} = 1 \times \dfrac{1760}{1} \times \dfrac{3}{1} \times \dfrac{12 \text{ in}}{1}$$

Step 5: Complete the required mathematical operations.

$$x \text{ in} = \dfrac{1 \times 1760 \times 3 \times 12 \text{ in}}{1 \times 1 \times 1} = 63{,}360 \text{ in}$$

Therefore, 63,360 inches = 1 mile.

Example 2.3: The previous problem could have been solved using two conversion factors as illustrated below.

Step 1: State the problem in equation form.

$x \text{ in} = 1 \text{ mile}$

Step 2: Identify the conversion factors needed to convert from miles to inches. Two conversion factors are needed:

A. Convert from miles to feet.

1 mile = 5280 feet gives $\dfrac{1 \text{ mile}}{5280 \text{ ft}}$ or $\dfrac{5280 \text{ ft}}{1 \text{ mile}}$

B. Convert from feet to inches.

1 foot = 12 inches gives $\dfrac{1 \text{ ft}}{12 \text{ in}}$ or $\dfrac{12 \text{ in}}{1 \text{ ft}}$

Step 3: Put into the equation the form of each conversion factor that will cancel the unwanted labels (miles and feet) and leave only the desired label (inches) on both sides of the equal sign.

$$x \text{ in} = 1 \text{ mile} \times \frac{5280 \text{ ft}}{1 \text{ mile}} \times \frac{12 \text{ in}}{1 \text{ ft}}$$

The equation can be read: x inches equal 1 mile when it is true that there are 5280 feet per 1 mile and when it is true that there are 12 inches per 1 foot.

Step 4: Cancel the labels that appear in both the numerator and the denominator on the same side of the equal sign.

$$x \text{ in} = 1 \times \frac{5280}{1} \times \frac{12 \text{ in}}{1}$$

Step 5: Complete the required mathematical operations.

$$x \text{ in} = \frac{1 \times 5280 \times 12 \text{ in}}{1 \times 1} = 63{,}360 \text{ in}$$

Therefore, 63,360 inches = 1 mile.

► SOLVED PRACTICE PROBLEMS

Conversion factors used to solve the problems in this exercise include:

12 inches = 1 foot	5280 feet = 1 mile
36 inches = 1 yard	16 ounces = 1 pound
3 feet = 1 yard	2000 pounds = 1 ton
1760 yards = 1 mile	

1. How many inches are equal to 3.5 feet?

$$x \text{ in} = 3.5 \text{ ft} \times \frac{12 \text{ in}}{1 \text{ ft}}$$

► **Answer:** 42 in

2. How many inches are equal to 4.25 yards?

$$x \text{ in} = 4.25 \text{ yd} \times \frac{3 \text{ ft}}{1 \text{ yd}} \times \frac{12 \text{ in}}{1 \text{ ft}}$$

► **Answer:** 153 in

3. How many feet are equal to 0.7 mile?

$$x \text{ ft} = 0.7 \text{ miles} \times \frac{5280 \text{ ft}}{1 \text{ mile}}$$

$$x \text{ ft} = 0.7 \text{ miles} \times \frac{1760 \text{ yd}}{1 \text{ mile}} \times \frac{3 \text{ ft}}{1 \text{ yd}}$$

► **Answer:** 3696 ft

4. How many inches are equal to 0.25 mile?

$$x \text{ in} = 0.25 \text{ mile} \times \frac{5280 \text{ ft}}{1 \text{ mile}} \times \frac{12 \text{ in}}{1 \text{ ft}}$$

$$x \text{ in} = 0.25 \text{ mile} \times \frac{1760 \text{ yd}}{1 \text{ mile}} \times \frac{3 \text{ ft}}{1 \text{ yd}} \times \frac{12 \text{ in}}{1 \text{ ft}}$$

▶ **Answer:** 15,840 in

5. How many ounces are equal to $3\frac{1}{2}$ pounds? *Note:* To simplify, use 3.5 pounds or 7/2 pounds.

$$x \text{ oz} = 3.5 \text{ lb} \times \frac{16 \text{ oz}}{1 \text{ lb}}$$

▶ **Answer:** 56 oz

6. How many ounces are equal to 0.0002 tons?

$$x \text{ oz} = 0.0002 \text{ ton} \times \frac{2000 \text{ lb}}{1 \text{ ton}} \times \frac{16 \text{ oz}}{1 \text{ lb}}$$

▶ **Answer:** 6.4 oz

▶ SELF-TEST

Express decimal answers to two decimal places.

1. How many yards are equal to 0.38 mile?
2. How many feet are equal to 0.0006 mile?
3. How many inches are equal to 0.0004 mile?
4. How many ounces are equal to 0.0005 ton?
5. How many ounces are equal to $6\frac{1}{4}$ pounds?
6. How many miles are equal to 2 million inches?
7. How many inches are equal to $3\frac{1}{5}$ yard?
8. How many pounds are equal to 1.35 tons?
9. How many tons are equal to 2000 ounces?
10. How many miles are in 5280 inches?

For answers to the self-test, see below.

---

1. 668.80 yd
2. 3.17 ft
3. 25.34 in
4. 16 oz
5. 100 oz

6. 31.57 miles
7. 115.20 in
8. 2700 lb
9. 0.06 tons
10. 0.08 miles

ANSWERS to Self-test

The Three Systems of Measurement

3

▲ OBJECTIVES

Upon completion of Chapter 3, the student will be able to:

- ► Recall the units, abbreviations, and symbols used in the metric, apothecary, and household systems of measurement.

- ► List the conversion factors (equivalents) used within the metric, apothecary, and household systems of measurement.

- ► Identify the conversion factors (equivalents) needed to convert from one system of measurement to another system of measurement.

- ► Apply the rules of problem solving by dimensional analysis to correctly calculate equivalent quantities within and among the three systems of measurement.

▲ THE METRIC SYSTEM

The metric system of measurement is the preferred system in the health sciences. At present it is the system of measurement used most widely in pharmacology. The majority of drugs are prescribed and dispensed in metric units. In order to use the metric system in dosage calculations, it is necessary that certain abbreviations, prefixes, and conversion factors (also called equivalents) be memorized (Table 3–1).

Converting among units of measurement in the metric system is easily accomplished by dimensional analysis. The five steps illustrated previously in Chapter 2 are used. Refer to Chapter 2 for review if needed.

Metric Calculations Requiring One Conversion Factor

Example 3.1 illustrates converting within the metric system using dimensional analysis. The example requires using only one conversion factor and involves working with simple fractions. It will be noted that converting units of dimensional analysis eliminates the need to move decimal places as a means of determining equivalents.

TABLE 3–1. METRIC UNITS AND CONVERSION FACTORS

Units of Measurement	Terminology of Prefixes	
Length	Kilo-	1000 times greater
m = meter	Centi-	100 times smaller
cm = centimeter	Milli-	1000 times smaller
mm = millimeter	Micro-	1,000,000 times smaller
Volume	*Conversion Factors/Equivalents*	
L = liter	1 m = 100 cm = 1000 mm	
ml = milliliter	1 L = 1000 ml = 1000 cc	
cc = cubic centimeter	1 kg = 1000 Gm	
Weight	1 Gm = 1000 mg	
kg = kilogram	1 mg = 1000 mcg	
Gm = gram	1 ml = 1 cc	
mg = milligram	Note: cc and ml are equivalent.	
mcg = microgram		
μg = microgram		

Example 3.1: How many grams are equal to 250 milligrams?

Step 1: State the problem in equation form.

$$x \, g \; = \; 250 \, mg$$

Step 2: Identify the conversion factor needed to convert from milligrams to grams: 1 g = 1000 mg.

Step 3. Put into the equation the form of the conversion factor that will cancel the unwanted label (milligrams) and leave only the desired label (grams) on both sides of the equal sign.

$$x \, g \; = \; 250 \, mg \; \times \; \frac{1 \, g}{1000 \, mg}$$

The equation can be read: *x* grams equal 250 milligrams when it is true that there is 1 gram per 1000 milligrams.

Step 4: Cancel the labels that appear in both the numerator and the denominator on the same side of the equal sign.

$$x \, g \; = \; 250 \; \times \; \frac{1 \, g}{1000}$$

Step 5: Complete the required mathematical operations.

$$x \, g \; = \; \frac{250 \times 1 \, g}{1000} \; = \; \frac{1 \times 1 \, g}{4} \; = \; 0.25 \, g$$

Therefore, 0.25 g = 250 mg.

Metric Calculations Requiring More Than One Conversion Factor

Examples 3.2 and 3.3 require working with more than one conversion factor. It will be necessary to put into each equation the form of *each conversion factor* that will cancel the unwanted labels from the equation.

Example 3.2: How many milligrams are in 2 kilograms?

Step 1: State the problem in equation form.

$$x \, mg \; = \; 2 \, kg$$

Step 2: Identify the conversion factors needed to convert from kilograms to milligrams. Two conversion factors are needed:

A. Convert from kilograms to grams.

1 kg = 1000 g

B. Convert from grams to milligrams.

1 g = 1000 mg

Step 3: Put into the equation the form of each conversion factor that will cancel the unwanted labels (kilograms and grams) and leave only the desired label (milligrams) on both sides of the equal sign.

$$x \, \text{mg} = 2 \, \text{kg} \times \frac{1000 \, \text{g}}{1 \, \text{kg}} \times \frac{1000 \, \text{mg}}{1 \, \text{g}}$$

The equation can be read: x milligrams equal 2 kilograms when it is true that there are 1000 grams per kilogram, and when it is true that there are 1000 milligrams per gram.

Step 4: Cancel the labels that appear in both the numerator and the denominator on the same side of the equal sign.

$$x \, \text{mg} = 2 \times \frac{1000}{1} \times \frac{1000 \, \text{mg}}{1}$$

Step 5: Complete the required mathematical operations.

$$x \, \text{mg} = \frac{2 \times 1000 \times 1000 \, \text{mg}}{1 \times 1} = 2{,}000{,}000 \, \text{mg}$$

Therefore, 2,000,000 mg = 2 kg.

Example 3.3: How many micrograms are equal to 0.0005 kilogram?

Step 1: State the problem in equation form.

$x \, \mu\text{g} = 0.0005 \, \text{kg}$

Step 2: Identify the conversion factors needed to convert from kilograms to micrograms. Three conversion factors are needed:

A. Convert from kilograms to grams.

1 kg = 1000 g

B. Convert from grams to milligrams.

1 g = 1000 mg

C. Convert from milligrams to micrograms.

1 mg = 1000 μg

Step 3: Put into the equation the form of each conversion factor that will cancel the unwanted labels (kilograms, grams, and milligrams) and leave only the desired label (micrograms) on both sides of the equal sign.

$$x \, \mu\text{g} = 0.0005 \, \text{kg} \times \frac{1000 \, \text{g}}{1 \, \text{kg}} \times \frac{1000 \, \text{mg}}{1 \, \text{g}} \times \frac{1000 \, \mu\text{g}}{1 \, \text{mg}}$$

The equation can be read: x micrograms equal 0.0005 kilograms when it is true that there are 1000 grams per 1 kilogram, and when it is true that there are 1000 milligrams per 1 gram, and when it is true that there are 1000 micrograms per 1 milligram.

Step 4: Cancel the labels that appear in both the numerator and the denominator on the same side of the equal sign.

$$x\,\mu g = 0.0005 \times \frac{1000}{1} \times \frac{1000}{1} \times \frac{1000\,\mu g}{1}$$

Step 5: Complete the required mathematical operations.

$$x\,\mu g = \frac{0.0005 \times 1000 \times 1000 \times 1000\,\mu g}{1 \times 1 \times 1} = 500{,}000\,\mu g$$

Therefore, 500,000 μg = 0.0005 kg.

► SOLVED PRACTICE PROBLEMS

1. How many grams are equal to 25 milligrams?

$$x\,g = 25\,mg \times \frac{1\,g}{1000\,mg}$$

► **Answer:** 0.025 g

2. How many micrograms are equal to 0.05 grams?

$$x\,\mu g = 0.05\,g \times \frac{1000\,mg}{1\,g} \times \frac{1000\,\mu g}{1\,mg}$$

► **Answer:** 50,000 μg

3. How many milligrams are equal to 0.2 kilograms?

$$x\,mg = 0.2\,kg \times \frac{1000\,g}{1\,kg} \times \frac{1000\,mg}{1\,g}$$

► **Answer:** 200,000 mg

4. How many micrograms are in 0.750 milligram?

$$x\,\mu g = 0.750\,mg \times \frac{1000\,\mu g}{1\,mg}$$

► **Answer:** 750 μg

5. How many milliliters are equal to 0.6 liter?

$$x\,ml = 0.6\,L \times \frac{1000\,ml}{1\,L}$$

► **Answer:** 600 ml

▲ APOTHECARY AND HOUSEHOLD EQUIVALENTS

The apothecary system is the original system of medication measurement used by pharmacists (apothecaries) and physicians. The system is still in use today to a limited extent (Table 3–2 and Figure 3–1). In general, drugs that continue to be ordered and dispensed in apothecary units are those that have been in use for many years. For most other drugs, the metric system is the system of measurement commonly used.

It is important to understand that the apothecary system is only approximately equivalent to the metric system and to the common household system of measurement. As a result, some of the equivalents relating the three systems are expressed as a range of values rather than single number values (Tables 3–3, 3–4, and 3–5).

In the apothecary system fractions and Roman numerals are commonly used to designate numbers. Morphine sulfate, for example, may be ordered as 1/4, 1/6, or 1/8 grain. In addition, atropine sulfate is frequently ordered as 1/150 grain or 1/200 grain. Roman numerals may or may not be capitalized and are often used in combination with "ss," which indicates 1/2. Therefore, the term iss means $1\frac{1}{2}$, and iiss means $2\frac{1}{2}$.

Remember

$$
\begin{array}{ll}
ss = 1/2 & iiiss = 3\frac{1}{2} \\
iss = 1\frac{1}{2} & ivss = 4\frac{1}{2} \\
iiss = 2\frac{1}{2} & vss = 5\frac{1}{2}
\end{array}
$$

TABLE 3–2. THE APOTHECARY SYSTEM OF MEASUREMENT

Abbreviations	Equivalents/Conversion Factors
Volume	
Minim = m	1 minim = 1 drop
Fluid dram = fl dr (ʒ)	1 fluid dram = 60 minims
Fluid ounce = fl oz (ʒ)	1 fluid ounce = 8 fluid drams
Weight	
Grain = gr	1 dram = 60 grains
Dram = dr	

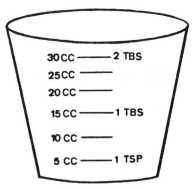 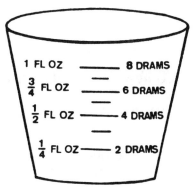

FIGURE 3–1. Medication cups with equivalent markings. (It can be noted in this figure that medication cups may be manufactured with the abbreviation, TBS, for tablespoon rather than the standard abbreviation, tbsp.)

TABLE 3–3. THE HOUSEHOLD SYSTEM OF MEASUREMENT

Abbreviations		Equivalents/Conversion Factors	
Volume			
Drop(s)	= gtt(s)	1 teaspoon	= 60 drops
Teaspoon	= tsp or t	1 tablespoon	= 3 teaspoons
Tablespoon	= tbsp or T	2 tablespoons	= 1 ounce
Ounce	= oz	1 cup	= 8 ounces
Pint	= pt	2 cups	= 1 pint
Quart	= qt	2 pints	= 1 quart
Gallon	= gal	4 quarts	= 1 gallon
Weight			
Pound	= lb	1 pound	= 16 ounces
Ounce	= oz		
Length			
Inch	= in	1 foot	= 12 inches
Foot	= ft		

TABLE 3–4. CONVERSION FACTORS/EQUIVALENTS

Household		Apothecary		Metric
Volume				
—	=	15–16 minims	=	1 milliliter
1 teaspoon	=	1 fluid dram	=	4–5 milliliters
1 tablespoon	=	3–4 fluid drams	=	15–16 milliliters
2 tablespoons	=	1 fluid ounce	=	30–32 milliliters
1 cup	=	8 fluid ounces	=	240 milliliters
1 pint	=	16 fluid ounces	=	500[a] milliliters
1 quart	=	32 fluid ounces	=	1000[a] milliliters
Weight				
—	=	1 grain	=	60–65 milligrams
—	=	15–16 grains	=	1 gram
—	=	1 dram	=	4 grams
2.2 pounds	=	—	=	1 kilogram
Length				
1 inch	=	—	=	2.54 centimeters
39.37 inches	=	—	=	1 meter

[a]In common practice these *approximate* equivalents are used.

TABLE 3–5. COMMONLY USED CONVERSION FACTORS

Volume	Weight
1 ml = 15 or 16 minims	1 gr = 60 or 64 mg
5 ml = 1 fl dr (ʒ) = 1 tsp	1 mg = 1000 mcg
15 ml = 4 fl dr (ʒ) = 1 tbsp	1 Gm = 1000 mg = 15 gr
30 ml = 8 fl dr (ʒ) = 1 oz (℥)	1 kg = 1000 Gm = 2.2 lb

▲ EQUIVALENTS RELATING THREE SYSTEMS OF MEASUREMENT

Converting within and Between Systems of Measurement

It is important to remember that when using the apothecary and household systems of measurement, several different conversion factors can often be used to solve the same problem. Due to the lack of precision of these systems, different conversion factors will often yield somewhat different answers. These answers, while different, would all be considered correct.

Example 3.4: How many milligrams are equal to grains vii?

Step 1: State the problem in equation form.

x mg = 7 gr

Step 2: Identify the conversion factor needed to convert from grains to milligrams: 1 gr = 60 mg.

Note: Since 1 gr = 60 to 65 mg, the problem could be solved using any one of the values from 60 to 65. The resulting answers, while different, would all be considered correct.

Step 3: Put into the equation the form of the conversion factor that will cancel the unwanted label (grains) and leave only the desired label (milligrams) on both sides of the equal sign.

$$x \text{ mg} = 7 \text{ gr} \times \frac{60 \text{ mg}}{1 \text{ gr}}$$

Step 4: Cancel the labels that appear in both the numerator and the denominator on the same side of the equal sign.

$$x \text{ mg} = 7 \times \frac{60 \text{ mg}}{1}$$

Step 5: Complete the required mathematical operations.

$$x \text{ mg} = \frac{7 \times 60 \text{ mg}}{1} = 420 \text{ mg}$$

Therefore, 420 mg = 7 gr.

Example 3.5: How many milligrams are equal to 0.2 pound?

Step 1: State the problem in equation form.

x mg = 0.2 lb

Step 2: Identify the conversion factors needed to convert from pounds to milligrams. Three conversion factors are needed:

A. Convert from pounds to kilograms.

2.2 lb = 1 kg

B. Convert from kilograms to grams.

1 kb = 1000 g

C. Convert from grams to milligrams.

1 g = 1000 mg

Step 3: Put into the equation the form of each conversion factor that will cancel the unwanted labels (pounds, kilograms, and grams) and leave only the desired label (milligrams) on both sides of the equal sign.

$$x \text{ mg} = 0.2 \text{ lb} \times \frac{1 \text{ kg}}{2.2 \text{ lb}} \times \frac{1000 \text{ g}}{1 \text{ kg}} \times \frac{1000 \text{ mg}}{1 \text{ g}}$$

Step 4: Cancel the labels that appear in both the numerator and the denominator on the same side of the equal sign.

$$x \text{ mg} = 0.2 \times \frac{1}{2.2} \times \frac{1000}{1} \times \frac{1000 \text{ mg}}{1}$$

Step 5: Complete the required mathematical operations.

$$x \text{ mg} = \frac{0.2 \times 1 \times 1000 \times 1000 \text{ mg}}{2.2 \times 1 \times 1} = 90{,}909 \text{ mg}$$

Therefore, 90,909 mg = 0.2 lb.

▶ SOLVED PRACTICE PROBLEMS

1. How many fluid ounces are equal to 16 fluid drams?

$$x \text{ fl dr} = 16 \text{ fl oz} \times \frac{1 \text{ fl oz}}{8 \text{ fl oz}}$$

▷ **Answer:** 2 fl oz

2. How many tablespoons are equal to 1/2 fluid ounce?

$$x \text{ tbsp} = \frac{1 \text{ fl oz}}{2} \times \frac{2 \text{ tbsp}}{1 \text{ fl oz}}$$

▷ **Answer:** 1 tbsp

3. How many milligrams are equal to grains ii?

$$x \text{ mg} = 2 \text{ gr} \times \frac{60 \text{ mg}}{1 \text{ gr}}$$

▷ **Answer:** 120 mg

4. How many minims are equal to 0.5 cubic centimeters?

$$x \text{ m} = 0.5 \text{ cc} \times \frac{15 \text{ m}}{1 \text{ cc}}$$

▷ **Answer:** 8 m

5. How many pounds are equal to 1200 grams?

$$x \text{ lb} = 1200 \text{ g} \times \frac{1 \text{ kg}}{1000 \text{ g}} \times \frac{2.2 \text{ lb}}{1 \text{ kg}}$$

▷ **Answer:** 2.64 lb

6. How many minims are equal to 3 fluid drams?

$$x \text{ m} = 3 \text{ fl dr} \times \frac{5 \text{ cc}}{1 \text{ fl dr}} \times \frac{15 \text{ m}}{1 \text{ cc}}$$

▷ **Answer:** 225 m

7. How many grams are equal to 2 ounces?

$$x \, g = 2 \, oz \times \frac{1 \, lb}{16 \, oz} \times \frac{1 \, kg}{2.2 \, lb} \times \frac{1000 \, g}{1 \, kg}$$

▷ **Answer:** 56.82 g

8. How many cubic centimeters are equal to $1\frac{1}{2}$ cups?

$$x \, cc = 1.5 \, cups \times \frac{8 \, oz}{1 \, cup} \times \frac{30 \, cc}{1 \, oz}$$

▷ **Answer:** 360 cc

9. How many milligrams are equal to 0.001 ounce?

$$x \, mg = 0.001 \, oz \times \frac{1 \, lb}{16 \, oz} \times \frac{1 \, kg}{2.2 \, lb} \times \frac{1000 \, g}{1 \, kg} \times \frac{1000 \, mg}{1 \, g}$$

▷ **Answer:** 28.41 mg

10. How many grains are equal to 0.0004 kilograms?

$$x \, gr = 0.0004 \, kg \times \frac{1000 \, g}{1 \, kg} \times \frac{15 \, gr}{1 \, g}$$

▷ **Answer:** 6 gr

Clinical Applications

Examples 3.6 and 3.7 illustrate clinical situations in which converting between systems of measurement is required. In these examples, the patient's fluid intake must be accurately measured and recorded. This is accomplished by converting all intake into a single unit of measure, the cubic centimeter.

Example 3.6: The physician ordered 8 ounces of Isocal (food supplement) to be given q4h by nasogastric tube to be followed by 50 cubic centimeters of water. In a 12 hour period, how many cubic centimeters of fluid would the patient receive?

Feeding q4h for 12 hours equals three feedings.

Part 1: Determine the number of cubic centimeters in one feeding. The conversion factor needed is: 1 oz = 30 cc.

$$x \, cc = 8 \, oz \times \frac{30 \, cc}{1 \, oz}$$

$$x \, cc = 240 \, cc$$

Therefore one feeding = 240 cc + 50 cc water. Total fluid in one feeding is *290 cc.*

Part 2:   Determine the total intake for 3 feedings. The conversion factor is: 1 feeding = 290 cc.

$$x \text{ cc} = 3 \text{ feedings} \times \frac{290 \text{ cc}}{1 \text{ feeding}}$$

$$x \text{ cc} = 870 \text{ cc}$$

Therefore, 870 cc is the *total* intake for *12 hours*.

Example 3.7: The patient is on strict intake and output measurement. Determine the fluid intake for a breakfast consisting of: $1\frac{1}{2}$ pints of milk, 6 ounces of juice, and $1\frac{1}{2}$ cups of coffee. With medications the patient drank 30 cubic centimeters of water.

Part 1:   How many cubic centimeters equal $1\frac{1}{2}$ pints of milk? (Using 1.5 is easier than $1\frac{1}{2}$ since it avoids using a mixed number.)

Conversion factor needed is: 1 pt = 500 cc

$$x \text{ cc} = 1.5 \text{ pt} \times \frac{500 \text{ cc}}{1 \text{ pt}}$$

$$x \text{ cc} = 750 \text{ cc}$$

Part 2:   How many cubic centimeters equal 6 ounces of juice?

Conversion factor needed is: 1 oz = 30 cc

$$x \text{ cc} = 6 \text{ oz} \times \frac{30 \text{ cc}}{1 \text{ oz}}$$

$$x \text{ cc} = 180 \text{ cc}$$

Part 3:   How many cubic centimeters equal $1\frac{1}{2}$ cups of coffee?

Conversion factor needed is: 1 cup = 240 cc

$$x \text{ cc} = 1.5 \text{ cups} \times \frac{240 \text{ cc}}{1 \text{ cup}}$$

$$x \text{ cc} = 360 \text{ cc}$$

Part 4:   Add: 750 cc milk + 180 cc juice + 360 cc coffee + 30 cc water

$$x \text{ cc} = 750 \text{ cc} + 180 \text{ cc} + 360 \text{ cc} + 30 \text{ cc}$$

Therefore, total intake is 1320 cc.

In Examples 3.8 and 3.9 length or height must be converted into centimeters. It is often necessary to express the weight or the length of an infant in metric units, since many growth charts are printed in metric units.

Example 3.8: A 3-month-old infant is found to have a head-to-foot length of 22 inches. Determine the length in centimeters.

Conversion factor needed is: 1 in = 2.54 cm.

$$x \text{ cm} = 22 \text{ in} \times \frac{2.54 \text{ cm}}{1 \text{ in}}$$

$$x \text{ cm} = 55.88 \text{ cm}$$

The total head-to-foot length = 55.88 cm.

Example 3.9: Find the height in centimeters of a child 3 feet tall.

Conversion factors needed are: 1 ft = 12 in, 1 in = 2.54 cm.

$$x \text{ cm} = 3 \text{ ft} \times \frac{12 \text{ in}}{1 \text{ ft}} \times \frac{2.54 \text{ cm}}{1 \text{ in}}$$

$$x \text{ cm} = 91.44 \text{ cm}$$

The child's height is 91.44 cm.

CASE STUDY

▸ Case One

Baby J., a 15-month-old toddler who weighs 22 pounds, 4 ounces, was admitted to the nursing unit with a diagnosis of dehydration. Among the physician's orders are the following: daily weight, I&O, weigh all diapers. During one 8-hour period the infant consumed $8\frac{1}{2}$ ounces of Pedialyte and two diapers were soiled with urine. The weight of wet diaper one was 130 grams and the weight of wet diaper two was 145 grams. The dry diapers weigh 92 grams each and each 1 milliliter of urine equals 1 gram.

Answer the following questions with reference to the case study:

1. What was the initial weight of the toddler in kilograms? (Express the answer to two decimal places.)
2. What was the intake of Pedialyte in milliliters?
3. What is the weight of a dry diaper?
4. What is the weight of the urine in diaper one?
5. What is the weight of the urine in diaper two?
6. What is the total weight of urine in both diapers?
7. What is the total urinary output of the toddler in milliliters?

For answers to the Case Study One, see page 51.

▸ SELF-TEST

Try to work the problems 3–20 with a minimum number of conversion factors. Remember that problems involving the apothecary and household systems of measurement can often be solved using several different conversion factors. The resulting answers may vary somewhat but would all be considered correct. For each of the problems in the self-test, only one possible answer is provided.

1. Supply the abbreviation or symbol:

   A. Dram _____   F. Gram _____

   B. Fluid dram _____   G. Milligram _____

   C. Fluid ounce _____ H. Teaspoon _____

   D. Grain _____   I. Tablespoon _____

   E. Minim _____

Continued next page

► **Self-Test Continued**

2. Supply the correct equivalent:

   A. 1 teaspoon   = _____ dram

   B. 1 tablespoon = _____ teaspoon

   C. 2 tablespoons = _____ ounce

   D. 1 gram   = _____ grain

   E. 60 milligrams = _____ grain

   F. 1 cup   = _____ ounce

   G. 1 milliliter = _____ minim

   H. 1 fluid dram = _____ milliliter

   I. 1 kilogram   = _____ pound

   J. 1 dram   = _____ gram

3. How many grams are equal to 20 drams?
4. How many milligrams are equal to 2 drams?
5. How many cc are equal to 2 fluid ounces?
6. How many grams are equal to 7 pounds, 4 ounces? First convert 4 ounces to pounds and express 7 pounds, 4 ounces as a number with a decimal.
7. What is the total intake in cubic centimeters if the patient drank 1/2 cup of coffee, 6 ounces of orange juice, 1 cup of milk, and 50 cubic centimeters of water with medications?
8. The physician ordered 4 ounces of Vivonex (food supplement) q2h followed by 10 cubic centimeters of water. In an 8 hour period, how many cubic centimeters of fluid does the patient receive?
9. How many kilograms are equal to 1/6 pound?
10. How many ounces are equal to 114 milligrams?
11. How many cups are equal to 128 ounces?
12. How many ounces are equal to 28.41 grams?
13. How many fluid drams are equal to 675 cubic centimeters?
14. How many grams are equal to grains viss?
15. How many tablespoons equal 45 cubic centimeters?
16. How many fluid drams are equal to 8.5 ounces?
17. How many centimeters are equal to 4 feet, 4 inches? (*Hint:* Convert 4 feet, 4 inches to the equivalent number of feet or inches before solving.)
18. How many feet are equal to 762 centimeters?
19. How many milliliters are equal to 5 teaspoons?
20. How many micrograms are equal to 0.0004 grams?

For answers to the self-test, see page 51.

1. 10.11 kg   4. 38 g   6. 91 g
2. 255 ml   5. 53 g   7. 91 ml
3. 92 g

1. See tables   8. 520 cc   15. 3 tbsp
2. See tables   9. 0.076 kg   16. 68 fl dr
3. 80 g   10. 0.004 oz   17. 132 cm
4. 8000 mg   11. 16 cups   18. 25 ft
5. 60 cc   12. 1 oz   19. 25 ml
6. 3295 g   13. 135 fl dr 20. 400 μg
7. 590 cc   14. 0.43 g

Nurse's Role in Drug Administration

4

▲ OBJECTIVES

Upon completion of Chapter 4, the student will be able to:

▸ Identify the legal components of a medication order.

▸ Understand the nurse's legal responsibilities in medication administration.

▸ Identify the "five rights" of medication administration.

▸ Correctly interpret information printed on drug labels.

Nurses are primarily responsible for the administration of prescribed medications to patients. This chapter presents information that will assist you in administering drugs correctly, ensuring that the patient receives the prescribed dose of the correct medication at the right time.

▲ COMPONENTS OF A LEGAL MEDICATION ORDER

In the inpatient setting, a medication order is written in the patient's chart on a specified order sheet identified with the patient's name, hospital ID number, and room number. The order is then processed and a medication administration record is generated either by computer or by hand. Figure 4–1 illustrates common components of a medication administration record.

Nurses administer medications in accordance with the orders written by health care provider licensed to prescribe medications. Licensed providers included physicians, dentists, nurse practitioners, and physician's assistants. A medication order written by a licensed provider must contain certain essential components to be considered a legal order. These components include:

1. Patient's name; and, for an inpatient, the patient's identification number.
2. Date the order is written; and, for an inpatient, the time the order is written.
3. The name of the drug (generic or trade) and dosage strength.

STATE UNIVERSITY MEDICAL CENTER

Yr: 97 Mon: 07		Day	1	2	3	4
Medication Name **Dose & Time**			**Initials** **Time**	**Initials** **Time**	**Initials** **Time**	**Initials** **Time**
Start date: *9/7/97* *Keflex p.o.* *500 mg q6h* **Discontinue:** *9/21/97*	i am i pm		mJm 6 + 12 Kaw 6-12	mJm 6 + 12 Kaw 6 - 12		
Start date: *9/7/97* *Sodium Heparin* *5000 U sc q12h* **Discontinue:**	i am i pm		mJm 9 Kaw 9	mJm 9 Kaw 9		
Start date: *9/7/97* *Lanoxin p.o.* *0.25 mg q am* **Discontinue:**	i am i pm		mJm 9	mJm 9		
Start date: *9/7/97* *Lasix p.o.* *20 mg b.i.d.* **Discontinue:**	i am i pm		9 5	9 5		

Initials	Signature	PATIENT IDENTIFICATION
mJm	Mary J Morgan	PAULINE M. JAMES # 33342141
Kaw	Ken A Wheeler	6001 23rd Street
		New Orleans, LA 70112

FIGURE 4–1.

4. Directions for administration, including the route and time interval or frequency; and, for an outpatient, length of time to take the drug.
5. The signature of the ordering provider; and, for outpatient prescriptions, the provider's licensing/DEA number.

▶ alert:

Any order is considered incomplete if it does not contain all the elements of an appropriate medication order.

▶ critical decision point:

The order reads: *Ativan 2 mg PO*
The order does not specify the time interval. The physician could have intended that one dose be given now and not again, but this is unclear.

▶ decision/action:

You determine that the order is ambiguous and call the physician to determine when the drug should be administered.

▲ MEDICATION NAMES AND LABELS

All drugs may be identified by both generic and trade names. The generic, or nonproprietary, name derives from the chemical substance from which the drug is made. This is the name approved by the Food and Drug Administration (FDA). The name *acetaminophen* is a generic name and, like all generic names, is spelled without a capital letter. The trade, or proprietary, name is the name given a drug by its manufacturer. The name *Tylenol* is a trade name registered for acetaminophen by a specific pharmaceutical company. The trade name is typically spelled with a capital letter. If a physician wants a particular trade name drug dispensed, the words "dispense as written" may appear in the drug order.

Medication labels generally contain the trade name of the drug in large print with the generic name generally printed below the trade name is smaller print. The label also indicates the form of the drug (e.g., tablets, capsules, elixir) and the strength of the drug.

Look at the label in Figure 4–2. The *trade name* of the drug is Lanoxin and the *generic name* is digoxin. The drug strength is 250 μg (0.25 mg) per tablet. Note that the tablets are scored so that they may be evenly divided into 125 μg (0.125 mg) doses.

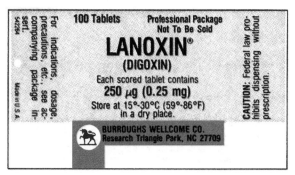

FIGURE 4–2.

In preparing medication for administration, the nurse must carefully read the medication label, checking the drug name and strength. In addition, the expiration date of the medication is checked to avoid administering a medication that has passed the expiration date. If a medication has passed its expiration date, it may have lost its potency or been chemically altered to produce a toxic drug form.

▲ EXERCISES

1. Study the label in Figure 4–3
   The generic name of the drug is _____
   The trade name of the drug is _____
   The strength of the drug is _____
   The drug form is _____

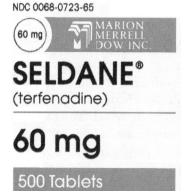
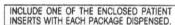

NDC 0068-0723-65

60 mg   MARION MERRELL DOW INC.

SELDANE®
(terfenadine)

60 mg

500 Tablets

H768B

INCLUDE ONE OF THE ENCLOSED PATIENT INSERTS WITH EACH PACKAGE DISPENSED.

Each tablet contains: terfenadine .... 60 mg

Usual Adult Dose: One tablet twice daily. See accompanying product information.

CAUTION: Federal law prohibits dispensing without prescription.

Keep tightly closed. Store at controlled room temperature 59-86°F (15-30°C).

Protect from exposure to temperatures above 104°F (40°C) and moisture.

Dispense in tight container with child-resistant closure.

©1995 Marion Merrell Dow Inc.
Manufactured by Marion & Company
Manati, PR 00674 for
Merrell Dow Pharmaceuticals Inc.
Subsidiary of
Marion Merrell Dow Inc.
Kansas City, MO 64114

FIGURE 4–3.

2. Study the label in Figure 4–4
   The generic name of the drug is _____
   The trade name of the drug is _____
   The strength of the drug is _____
   The drug form is _____

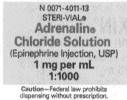

N 0071-4011-13
STERI-VIAL®
Adrenalin®
Chloride Solution
(Epinephrine Injection, USP)
1 mg per mL
1:1000

Caution—Federal law prohibits dispensing without prescription.

30 mL

® PARKE-DAVIS
People Who Care

FIGURE 4–4.

3. Study the label in Figure 4–5
   The generic name of the drug is _____
   The trade name of the drug is _____
   The strength of the drug is _____
   The drug form is _____

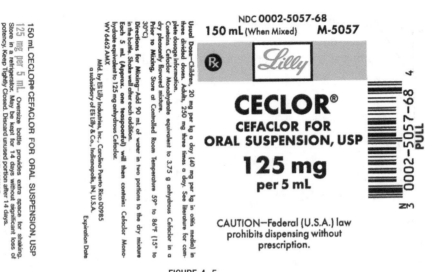

FIGURE 4–5.

4. Study the label in Figure 4–6
   The generic name of the drug is _____
   The trade name of the drug is _____
   The strength of the drug is _____
   The drug form is _____

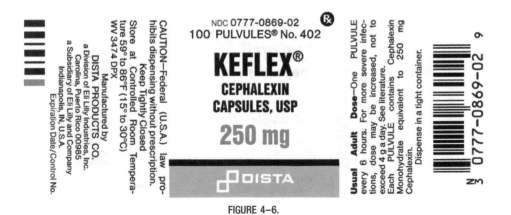

FIGURE 4–6.

Answers: Figure 4–3: terfenadine; Seldane; 60 mg; tablet
Figure 4–4: epinephrine; Adrenalin; 1 mg per ml; liquid for injection
Figure 4–5: cefaclor, Ceclor; 125 mg per 5 ml; oral suspension
Figure 4–6: cephalexin; Keflex; 250 mg; capsules or pulvules

▲ NURSES' LEGAL RESPONSIBILITIES

The nurse is legally responsible for correctly administering medications to patients. To interpret the physician's order correctly, the nurse must be knowledgeable about types of pharmaceutical preparations, their actions, usual dosages, methods of administration, and common abbreviations and symbols used in medications orders (see Appendix A). Areas of potential confusion related to the medication order include:

1. Illegible words, numbers, or symbols
2. Unusual abbreviations or symbols
3. Misspelled words or drug names
4. Unreasonable doses
5. Unusual times or frequencies for administration

► alert:

If the physician's order seems out of the ordinary, you must question the order.

► critical decision point:

The order reads: *Give 750 mg of Ludiomil q.d.*
You check the medication label (see Figure 4–7) and find that the medication is supplied in 75 mg tablets. You determine that a 750 mg dose would require 10 tablets. You check the **Nurses Drug Guide** and find the normal dose is 75 mg q.d.

► decision/action:

You decide that the ordered dose is much greater than the usual dose. You call the physician to clarify the dose.

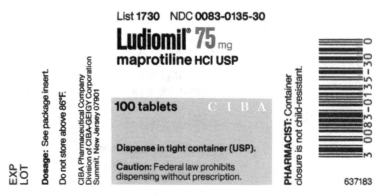

FIGURE 4–7.

Five Rights of Medication Administration

The legal responsibilities of the nurse are often summarized as the five rights of medication administration. These summarize the nurse's responsibilities in medication administration. When implemented correctly, these five rights eliminate common sources of medication errors. The five rights are:

1. The right patient
2. The right drug

3. The right dose
4. The right route
5. The right time

All of the information needed for the five rights is specified in the medication order. It is the nurse's responsibility to check this information as the drug is prepared for administration.

- **The Right Patient:** In the inpatient setting, always double-check the patient's name band. The nurse cannot assume that a patient answering in the affirmative when a name is called is the right patient.
- **The Right Drug:** Check the drug name carefully, because many drugs have similar-sounding names, similar spelling, or similar-looking labels. Examples of names that could be easily confused are: Zantac and Xanax; cefotetan and cefotaxime. There are many other similar examples; therefore, if an order is difficult to read, the nurse should **not attempt to guess** what the prescriber intended.
- **The Right Route:** Medications are manufactured to be administered by a specific route. The ordered route should be carefully checked as many medications may be administered by several different routes. When given by the incorrect route, the medication could be ineffective or even toxic.
- **The Right Time:** Medications are ordered either on a regular schedule or prn. A prn order indicates that the medication may be given at certain intervals if needed. Scheduled medications are given as ordered unless some untoward event occurs. An order may specify the administration time generally or quite specifically. For example, a drug may be ordered "q.d." (one a day) or "q AM" (every morning). In the inpatient setting, institutional policy will most often dictate standard times for drug administration. The nurse is responsible for administering medications as ordered according to institutional policy.
- **The Right Dose:** The nurse is not only responsible for administering the ordered dose but also for determining that the ordered dose is appropriate. The nurse should ask what the recommended dose is for this drug and if the ordered dose is appropriate for this patient. It is the nurse's legal responsibility to administer only appropriate doses. If a nurse is not certain of the recommended dose of a particular drug, the nurse must determine this information by using an appropriate reference prior to administering the drug.

▸ alert:

A drug order may be missing one element, which may be overlooked by the nurse. Do not assume you know what the missing element is.

▸ critical decision point:

The order reads: *Chewable Tegretol PO b.i.d.*
You find two different strengths of Tegretol in the medication cart, each with the labels indicated in Figure 4–8. The order is ambiguous since it does not specify dose.

action:

You cannot assume that the 100 mg dose is intended just because this is a chewable form. You must call the physician for clarification of the ordered dose.

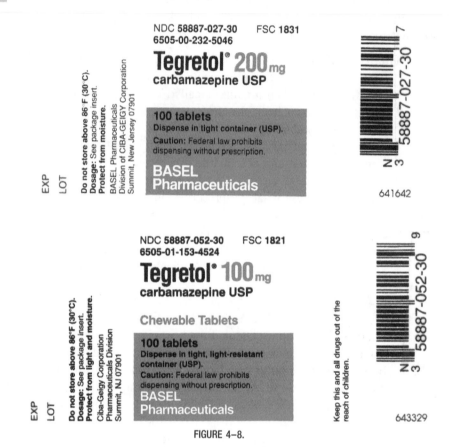

FIGURE 4–8.

▲ COMMON MEDICATION ERRORS

The most common medication errors stem from inadequate attention to the five rights of medication administration. Common errors include the following:

- **Wrong Patient:** In the inpatient setting, the nurse may administer a medication to the roommate of the intended patient because of inattentiveness to patient identification arm bands.
- **Wrong Drug:** The nurse may pick a medication that appears to be correct without double-checking the actual name of the drug. For example: giving NPH insulin rather than regular insulin.
- **Wrong Route:** A common error is misadministration of an oral form of a drug. For example, a chewable tablet is swallowed whole or a sustained-action tablet is chewed or crushed.
- **Wrong Time:** Errors in time occur when nurses administer medications later or earlier than scheduled. In either case, when this occurs drugs could be given concurrently that inactivate one another. A common mistake in this regard is giving antacids with other medications which were ordered to be given 1–2 hours before the antacid.

- **Wrong Dose:** The wrong dose may be given by oversight such as failure to double-check the dose indicated on the drug label. Study Figure 4–9. Note that the labels look exactly alike except for the strength (7.5 mg or 15 mg) and the color of the bar under the strength (yellow and blue, respectively). Another common error is a mistaken drug calculation. A nurse who is unsure of a calculation should always have a colleague verify the calculation.

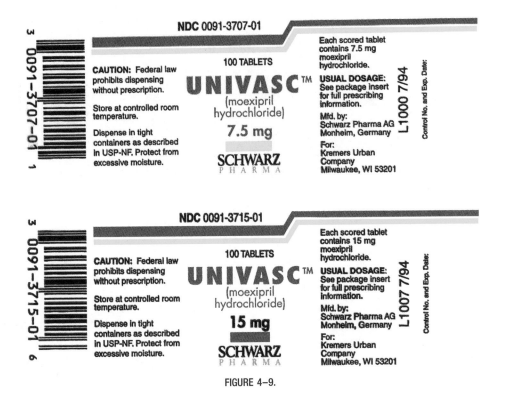

FIGURE 4–9.

Nonparenteral Medications

5

▲ OBJECTIVES

Upon completion of Chapter 5, the student will be able to:

- ► Express the numerical value of the amount of medication to be administered in clinically feasible quantities using either solid or liquid forms of medication.

- ► Apply the rules of problem solving by dimensional analysis to calculations involving nonparenteral medications.

- ► Correctly calculate the number of tablets, pills, capsules, or suppositories needed to administer the prescribed dose using in the calculations one or more conversion factors and simple or complex fractions.

- ► Correctly calculate the number of ounces, teaspoons, tablespoons, drams, or milliliters needed to administer the prescribed dose using in the calculations one or more conversion factors and simple or complex fractions.

- ► Correctly calculate the amount of medication needed to last a specified amount of time.

- ► Correctly calculate how many days or doses a given quantity of medication will last.

▲ INTRODUCTION TO NONPARENTERAL MEDICATIONS

This chapter deals with nonparenteral medications. Nonparenteral medications include those given in the following ways: oral, topical, rectal, and vaginal. Oral medications are frequently prescribed and easy to administer. Drugs given by this route usually have systemic effects; however, some oral medications have specific sites of action.

Oral medications are dispensed in a variety of forms. Among the more common forms that require drug calculations are:

1. Tablets: Made by compression and molding of medical substances; produced without a coating in scored and unscored forms; scored forms may be broken in order to administer half a tablet

2. Capsules: Solid dosage form enclosed within a gelatin container
3. Pills: Coated tablets that are not scored
4. Elixirs: Drug preparations dissolved in a solution of alcohol and water; a tincture has a higher alcohol content
5. Suspensions: Finely divided drugs held in suspension in a liquid medium; they must be shaken before administration
6. Syrups: Drug preparation dissolved in water and sugar

exercise

▲ NONPARENTERAL DRUG FORMS

Solid Preparations: Information regarding the strength of solid forms of medication is printed on the drug label. Typically, other important information may be found on the label. Refer to the Procan SR label in Figure 5–1 to answer the following questions:

1. What is the generic name for Procan?
2. What is the strength of each Procan tablet?
3. What is the meaning of the designation "SR" after the name?
4. What special direction should be given to the patient about swallowing this drug?
5. How should the drug be stored?

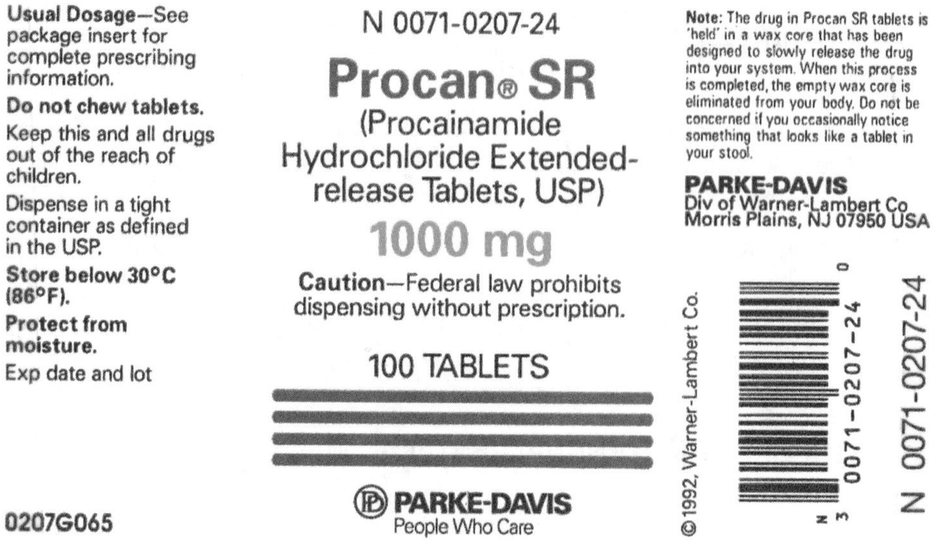

Usual Dosage—See package insert for complete prescribing information.

Do not chew tablets.

Keep this and all drugs out of the reach of children.

Dispense in a tight container as defined in the USP.

Store below 30°C (86°F).

Protect from moisture.

Exp date and lot

0207G065

N 0071-0207-24

Procan® SR
(Procainamide Hydrochloride Extended-release Tablets, USP)

1000 mg

Caution—Federal law prohibits dispensing without prescription.

100 TABLETS

Ⓟ **PARKE-DAVIS**
People Who Care

Note: The drug in Procan SR tablets is 'held' in a wax core that has been designed to slowly release the drug into your system. When this process is completed, the empty wax core is eliminated from your body. Do not be concerned if you occasionally notice something that looks like a tablet in your stool.

PARKE-DAVIS
Div of Warner-Lambert Co
Morris Plains, NJ 07950 USA

© 1992, Warner-Lambert Co.

N 0071-0207-24

FIGURE 5–1.

Answers: procainamide hydrochloride; 1000 mg; slow release; do not chew; below 30C/86F and protected from moisture

Liquid Preparations: Information regarding the concentration of an oral liquid or suspension is printed on the drug label. Typically, other important information may be found on the label. Refer to the Vistaril label in Figure 5–2.

1. What is the concentration of the Vistaril suspension?
2. One teaspoon of Vistaril contains how many milligrams (mg) of medication?
3. How many milliliters (ml) equal one teaspoon of Vistaril?
4. Prior to pouring this drug for administration, what should you do?
5. What is the maximum temperature at which Vistaril can be stored?

NDC 0069-5440-93

Vistaril®
(hydroxyzine pamoate)

ORAL SUSPENSION

*Each teaspoonful (5mL) contains
hydroxyzine pamoate equivalent
to 25 mg hydroxyzine hydrochloride.

USUAL DAILY DOSAGE
Adults: 1 to 4 teaspoonfuls 3-4 times daily
Children: 6 years and over–2 to 4 teaspoonfuls
daily in divided doses.
Under 6 years–2 teaspoonfuls daily
in divided doses.

**READ ACCOMPANYING
PROFESSIONAL INFORMATION.**

Store below 77°F (25°C)

Dispense in tight, light-resistant containers (USP)

**SHAKE VIGOROUSLY UNTIL PRODUCT IS
COMPLETELY RESUSPENDED.**

IMPORTANT: This closure is not child-resistant

DYE FREE FORMULA

| **CAUTION:** Federal law prohibits dispensing without prescription. | 05-0844-00-4 MADE IN USA 4387 |

1 Pint (473 mL)

Vistaril®
(hydroxyzine pamoate)

E005A
EXP 1 MAY 00

ORAL SUSPENSION

25 mg/5 mL*

For Oral Use Only

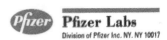

3 0069-5440-93 9

Pfizer **Pfizer Labs**
Division of Pfizer Inc. NY, NY 10017

FIGURE 5–2.

Answers: 25 mg/5 ml; 25 mg; 5 ml; shake vigorously; 25C/77F

► alert:

Only scored tablets can be accurately broken into known quantities.

► critical decision point:

The order reads: *isosorbide mononitrate 10 mg PO and Lopressor 50 mg PO.*
The available form of isosorbide mononitrate is Monoket, which is labeled as

indicated in Figure 5–3. The Monoket label indicates that each tablet is a deep-scored 20 mg tablet. The available form of Lopressor is labeled as indicated in Figure 5–4. The Lopressor label indicates that each tablet is 100 mg. You inspect the tablets and find they are not scored.

► decision/action:

The Monoket tablet may be broken in half to provide a 10 mg dose. The Lopressor tablets should not be broken since you cannot ensure that the 100 mg tablet will be broken evenly into two 50 mg parts. You should contact the pharmacists to obtain the correct dosage form of Lopressor.

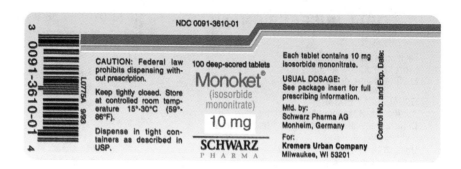

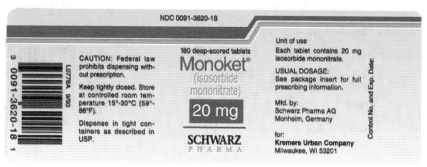

FIGURE 5–3.

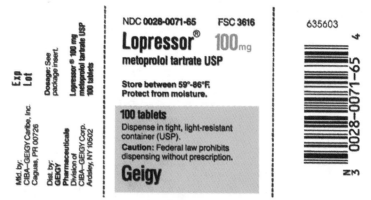

FIGURE 5–4.

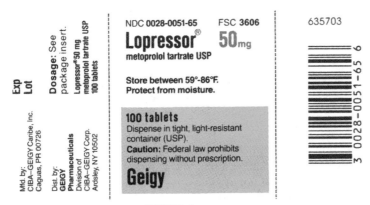

FIGURE 5–4.

▲ CALCULATING DOSAGE OF NONPARENTERAL MEDICATIONS

All calculations in this unit on nonparenteral medications are carried out using the dimensional analysis method of problem solving discussed in Chapter 2. In Example 5.1, the application of the method to dosage calculations is illustrated.

Rounding answers. Answers to problems involving pills, capsules, and *unscored* tablets or suppositories should be rounded to the nearest *whole* number. *Scored* tablets or suppositories should be rounded to the nearest *half*. With problems involving oral, liquid medications, it is generally accurate enough to round to one decimal place. Medications for infants and small children may require a greater degree of accuracy.

Example 5.1: How many tablets would you administer if the doctor ordered 2 mg of Ativan (lorazepam)? Available are 0.5 mg tablets.

▶ Rules of Problem Solving by Dimensional Analysis

 One side of an equation can be multiplied by an appropriate conversion factor without changing the value of the equation.

◀ RULE 1

▶ Application of Rule 1

In all medication calculations, the dosage form in which the drug is manufactured is considered to be a conversion factor. In the example given above, one tablet of Ativan contains 0.5 milligrams of medication. Therefore, the conversion factor (1 tab = 0.5 mg) can be put into the problem in either of two possible forms:

$$\frac{1 \text{ tab}}{0.5 \text{ mg}} \quad \text{or} \quad \frac{0.5 \text{ mg}}{1 \text{ tab}}$$

 The problem is correctly set up when all labels cancel from both the numerator and denominator except the label that is desired in the answer.

◀ RULE 2

► Application of Rule 2

1. In the problem given, the question asked is how many tablets of Ativan equal a 2 milligram dose.
2. Stated in an equation form, the problem is

x tab $= 2$ mg

3. The conversion factor, 1 tab $= 0.5$ mg, is put into the equation as a fraction. The form of the fraction used is that which will cancel the unwanted label (milligrams) and leave only the desired label (tablets) on both sides of the equal sign.

$$x \text{ tab } = 2 \text{ mg } \times \frac{1 \text{ tab}}{0.5 \text{ mg}}$$

The equation can be read: x tablets equal 2 milligrams when it is true that 1 tablet contains 0.5 milligrams.

4. Cancel labels that appear in both the numerator and denominator on the *same* side of the equal sign.

$$x \text{ tab } = 2 \times \frac{1 \text{ tab}}{0.5}$$

5. Complete the required mathematical operations.

$$x \text{ tab } = \frac{2 \times 1 \text{ tab}}{0.5} = 4 \text{ tab}$$

Therefore, four 0.5 mg tablets of Ativan will provide the ordered dose.

The method of problem solving by dimensional analysis illustrated above is used throughout this unit.

One Conversion Factor and Simple Fractions

Examples 5.2 and 5.3, which follow, are similar to Example 5.1. Each of these examples requires using only one conversion factor and involves working with simple fractions.

Example 5.2: The physician has ordered 600,000 units of V-cillin K (penicillin V) per dose. On hand are 400,000 unit tablets. How many scored tablets should you give?

Step 1: State the problem in equation form.

x tab $= 600,000$ U

Step 2: Identify the conversion factor needed to convert from units to tablets: 1 tab $= 400,000$ U.

Step 3: Put into the equation the form of the conversion factor that will cancel the unwanted label (units) and leave only the desired label (tablets) on both sides of the equal sign.

$$x \text{ tab } = 600,000 \text{ U } \times \frac{1 \text{ tab}}{400,000 \text{ U}}$$

Step 4: Cancel the labels that appear in both the numerator and the denominator on the same side of the equal sign.

$$x \, \text{tab} = 600,000 \times \frac{1 \, \text{tab}}{400,000}$$

Step 5: Complete the required mathematical operations.

$$x \, \text{tab} = 1\tfrac{1}{2} \, \text{tab}$$

Therefore, $1\tfrac{1}{2}$ tablets will provide the ordered dose. Note that scored tablets can be divided evenly in half.

Example 5.3: The physician's order is to give the patient $1\tfrac{1}{2}$ fl dr of Organidin (iodinated glycerol) prn. How many cc will you give?

Step 1: State the problem in equation form.

$$x \, \text{cc} = 1\tfrac{1}{2} \, \text{fl dr}$$

Change the mixed number ($1\tfrac{1}{2}$) to a decimal (1.5) or an improper fraction (3/2) to solve the problem.

$$x \, \text{cc} = 1.5 \, \text{fl dr}$$

Step 2: Identify the conversion factor needed to convert from fluid dram to cubic centimeters: 1 fl dr = 5 cc.

Step 3: Put into the equation the form of the conversion factor that will cancel the unwanted label and leave only the desired label on both sides of the equal sign.

$$x \, \text{cc} = 1.5 \, \text{fl dr} \times \frac{5 \, \text{cc}}{1 \, \text{fl dr}}$$

Step 4: Cancel the labels that appear in both the numerator and the denominator on the same side of the equal sign.

$$x \, \text{cc} = 1.5 \times \frac{5 \, \text{cc}}{1}$$

Step 5: Complete the required mathematical operations.

$$x \, \text{cc} = 7.5 \, \text{cc}$$

Therefore, 7.5 cc will provide the ordered dose.

► SOLVED PRACTICE PROBLEMS

1. The order is to give Ritalin (methylphenidate) 30 mg PO b.i.d. On hand are 20-mg tablets. How many scored tablets will you give?

$$x \, \text{tablet} = 30 \, \text{mg} \times \frac{1 \, \text{tab}}{20 \, \text{mg}}$$

► **Answer:** $1\tfrac{1}{2}$ tablets

2. The order is to give 875 mg of Mysoline (primidone) PO q.i.d. On hand are 250-mg tablets. How many scored tablets will you give?

$$x \text{ tab} = 875 \text{ mg} \times \frac{1 \text{ tab}}{250 \text{ mg}}$$

▸ **Answer:** $3\frac{1}{2}$ tablets

3. The order is to give 500 mg of ampicillin suspension PO q6h. The available suspension contains 125 mg per 5 cc. How many cc will you give?

$$x \text{ cc} = 500 \text{ mg} \times \frac{5 \text{ cc}}{125 \text{ mg}}$$

▸ **Answer:** 20 cc

4. The order is to give 100 mg of Dilantin (phenytoin) orally t.i.d. The available suspension contains 30 mg per 5 cc. How many cc will you give?

$$x \text{ cc} = 100 \text{ mg} \times \frac{5 \text{ cc}}{30 \text{ mg}}$$

▸ **Answer:** 16.7 cc; therefore give 17 cc

5. The order is to give tetracycline syrup, 375 mg q6h PO. The available medication contains 125 mg per tsp. How many tsp will you give?

$$x \text{ tsp} = 375 \text{ mg} \times \frac{1 \text{ tsp}}{125 \text{ mg}}$$

▸ **Answer:** 3 tsp

One Conversion Factor and Complex Fractions

A complex fraction has either a mixed number or a fraction in the numerator, denominator, or both. Two examples of complex fractions are given below:

1. Fraction in the numerator

$$\frac{\dfrac{1 \text{ gr}}{8}}{1 \text{ cap}}$$

2. Fraction in the denominator

$$\frac{1 \text{ tab}}{\dfrac{1 \text{ gr}}{3}}$$

Working with complex fractions is more convenient if they are first simplified. To simplify a complex fraction, it is necessary to invert the denominator, and then multiply the numerator by the denominator. This procedure, referred to as invert and multiply, is used to simplify the complex fractions in Examples 5.4 and 5.5, which follow.

Example 5.4: How many tablets of Amytal (amobarbital) will you administer if the physician orders 1/6 gr and you have available 1/3 gr scored tablets?

Step 1: State the problem in equation form.

$$x\,\text{tab} = \frac{1\,\text{gr}}{6}$$

Step 2: Identify the conversion factor needed to convert from grains to tablets: 1 tab = 1/3 gr.

Step 3: Put into the equation the form of the conversion factor that will cancel the unwanted label and leave only the desired label on both sides of the equal sign.

$$x\,\text{tab} = \frac{1\,\text{gr}}{6} \times \frac{1\,\text{tab}}{\dfrac{1\,\text{gr}}{3}}$$

The steps used to simplify the complex fraction are illustrated below:

A. $\dfrac{1\,\text{tab}}{\dfrac{1\,\text{gr}}{3}}$ is the same as $1\,\text{tab} \div \dfrac{1\,\text{gr}}{3}$

B. Invert and multiply to get: $1\,\text{tab} \times \dfrac{3}{1\,\text{gr}}$

C. Substitute the simplified form of the expression into the equation in place of the complex fraction.

Therefore: $1\,\text{tab} \times \dfrac{3}{1\,\text{gr}}$ replaces $\dfrac{1\,\text{tab}}{\dfrac{1\,\text{gr}}{3}}$

$$x\,\text{tab} = \frac{1\,\text{gr}}{6} \times 1\,\text{tab} \times \frac{3}{1\,\text{gr}}$$

Step 4: Cancel the labels that appear in both the numerator and the denominator on the same side of the equal sign.

$$x\,\text{tab} = \frac{1}{6} \times 1\,\text{tab} \times \frac{3}{1}$$

Step 5: Complete the required mathematical operations.

$$x\,\text{tab} = 1/2\,\text{tab}$$

Therefore, 1/2 tablet will provide the ordered dose.

Example 5.5: The patient is to receive an analgesic cocktail solution that contains 1/4 gr morphine per 5 cc. How many gr of morphine would be contained in 4 cc of the cocktail?

Step 1: State the problem in equation form.

$$x\,\text{gr} = 4\,\text{cc}$$

Step 2: Identify the conversion factor needed to convert from cubic centimeters to grains: 5 cc = 1/4 gr.

Step 3: Put into the equation the form of the conversion factor that will cancel the unwanted label and leave only the desired label on both sides of the equal sign.

$$x \text{ gr} = 4 \text{ cc} \times \frac{\frac{1 \text{ gr}}{4}}{5 \text{ cc}}$$

The steps used to simplify the complex fraction are illustrated below:

A. $\dfrac{\frac{1 \text{ gr}}{4}}{5 \text{ cc}}$ is the same as: $\dfrac{1 \text{ gr}}{4} \div 5 \text{ cc}$

B. Invert and multiply to get: $\dfrac{1 \text{ gr}}{4} \times \dfrac{1}{5 \text{ cc}}$

C. Substitute the simplified form of the expression into the equation in place of the complex fraction.

Therefore: $\dfrac{1 \text{ gr}}{4} \times \dfrac{1}{5 \text{ cc}}$ replaces $\dfrac{\frac{1 \text{ gr}}{4}}{5 \text{ cc}}$

$$x \text{ gr} = 4 \text{ cc} \times \frac{1 \text{ gr}}{4} \times \frac{1}{5 \text{ cc}}$$

Step 4: Cancel the labels that appear in both the numerator and the denominator on the same side of the equal sign.

$$x \text{ gr} = 4 \times \frac{1 \text{ gr}}{4} \times \frac{1}{5}$$

Step 5: Complete the required mathematical operations.

$$x \text{ gr} = \frac{1 \text{ gr}}{5}$$

Therefore, 4 cc contains 1/5 grain of morphine.

▶ SOLVED PRACTICE PROBLEMS

1. The order is to give atropine 1/100 gr PO q6h. On hand are scored 1/150 gr tablets. How many tablets will you give?

$$x \text{ tab} = \frac{1 \text{ gr}}{100} \times \frac{1 \text{ tab}}{\frac{1 \text{ gr}}{150}}$$

Simplified: $x \text{ tab} = \dfrac{1 \text{ gr}}{100} \times 1 \text{ tab} \times \dfrac{150}{1 \text{ gr}}$

▶ **Answer:** $1\frac{1}{2}$ tablets

2. The order is to give morphine 1/4 gr PO stat. On hand are scored 1/2 gr tablets. How many tablets would you give?

$$x \text{ tab} = \frac{1 \text{ gr}}{4} \times \frac{1 \text{ tab}}{\dfrac{1 \text{ gr}}{2}}$$

Simplified: $x \text{ tab} = \dfrac{1 \text{ gr}}{4} \times 1 \text{ tab} \times \dfrac{2}{1 \text{ gr}}$

▶ **Answer:** 1/2 tablet

3. The order is to give 3/8 gr of phenobarbital PO prn for agitation. On hand are scored 1/4-gr tablets. How many tablets would you give?

$$x \text{ tab} = \frac{3 \text{ gr}}{8} \times \frac{1 \text{ tab}}{\dfrac{1 \text{ gr}}{4}}$$

Simplified: $x \text{ tab} = \dfrac{3 \text{ gr}}{8} \times 1 \text{ tab} \times \dfrac{4}{1 \text{ gr}}$

▶ **Answer:** $1\frac{1}{2}$ tablets

4. The order is to give B & O supprettes (belladonna and opium) gr 3/4 prn q6h for discomfort. On hand are gr 1/2 supprettes. How many will you give? The supprettes are scored for even division.

$$x \text{ supp} = \frac{3 \text{ gr}}{4} \times \frac{1 \text{ supp}}{\dfrac{1 \text{ gr}}{2}}$$

Simplified: $x \text{ supp} = \dfrac{3 \text{ gr}}{4} \times 1 \text{ supp} \times \dfrac{2}{1 \text{ gr}}$

▶ **Answer:** $1\frac{1}{2}$ supprettes

5. The order is to give thyroid extract gr $1\frac{1}{2}$. On hand are 1/4-gr tablets. How many scored tablets will you give?

$$x \text{ tab} = 1.5 \text{ gr} \times \frac{1 \text{ tab}}{\dfrac{1 \text{ gr}}{4}}$$

Simplified: $x \text{ tab} = 1.5 \text{ gr} \times 1 \text{ tab} \times \dfrac{4}{1 \text{ gr}}$

▶ **Answer:** 6 tablets

More than One Conversion Factor

Examples 5.6 and 5.7 require working with more than one conversion factor. It will be necessary to put into each equation the form of *each* conversion factor that will cancel the unwanted labels from the equation.

Example 5.6: The physician ordered gr X Tylenol (acetaminophen) elixir q4h prn for temperature elevation greater than 101F. The elixir contains 120 mg per 5 cc. How many cc will you give?

Step 1: State the problem in equation form.

x cc $= 10$ gr

Step 2: Identify the conversion factors needed to convert from grains to cubic centimeters. Two conversion factors are used:

A. Convert from grains to milligrams.

1 gr $= 60$ mg

B. Convert from milligrams to cubic centimeters.

120 mg $= 5$ cc

Step 3: Put into the equation the form of each conversion factor that will cancel the unwanted labels and leave only the desired label on both sides of the equal sign.

$$x \text{ cc} = 10 \text{ gr} \times \frac{60 \text{ mg}}{1 \text{ gr}} \times \frac{5 \text{ cc}}{120 \text{ mg}}$$

Step 4: Cancel the labels that appear in both the numerator and the denominator on the same side of the equal sign.

$$x \text{ cc} = 10 \times \frac{60}{1} \times \frac{5 \text{ cc}}{120}$$

Step 5: Complete the required mathematical operations.

x cc $= 25$ cc

Therefore, 25 cc will provide the ordered dose.

Example 5.7: How many tsp of Lanoxin (digoxin) pediatric elixir would you give if the order is 0.25 mg q AM? The elixir available contains 50 μg per 1 ml.

Step 1: State the problem in equation form.

x tsp $= 0.25$ mg

Step 2: Identify the conversion factors needed to convert from milligrams to teaspoons. Three conversion factors are used:

A. Convert from milligrams to micrograms.

1 mg $= 1000$ μg

B. Convert from micrograms to milliliters.

50 μg $= 1$ ml

C. Convert from milliliters to teaspoons.

5 ml $= 1$ tsp

Step 3: Put into the equation the form of each conversion factor that will cancel the unwanted labels and leave only the desired label on both sides of the equal sign.

$$x \text{ tsp} = 0.25 \text{ mg} \times \frac{1000 \text{ } \mu g}{1 \text{ mg}} \times \frac{1 \text{ ml}}{50 \text{ } \mu g} \times \frac{1 \text{ tsp}}{5 \text{ ml}}$$

Step 4:   Cancel the labels that appear in both the numerator and the denominator on the same side of the equal sign.

$$x \text{ tsp} = 0.25 \times \frac{1000}{1} \times \frac{1}{50} \times \frac{1 \text{ tsp}}{5}$$

Step 5:   Complete the required mathematical operations.

$$x \text{ tsp} = 1 \text{ tsp}$$

Therefore, 1 teaspoon will provide the ordered dose.

▶ SOLVED PRACTICE PROBLEMS

1. The physician ordered 1/2 fl oz of Milk of Magnesia. How many tsp will you give?

$$x \text{ tsp} = \frac{1 \text{ fl oz}}{2} \times \frac{30 \text{ cc}}{1 \text{ fl oz}} \times \frac{1 \text{ tsp}}{5 \text{ cc}}$$

▶ **Answer:**   3 tsp

2. The physician ordered phenobarbital gr ss in elixir form q6h. The label states that there are 20 mg per 5 ml of the medication. How many cc will you give?

$$x \text{ cc} = \frac{1 \text{ gr}}{2} \times \frac{60 \text{ mg}}{1 \text{ gr}} \times \frac{5 \text{ cc}}{20 \text{ mg}}$$

▶ **Answer:**   7.5 cc

3. The order is for Amytal (amobarbital) 60 mg PO. On hand are capsules labeled gr 1/4. How many capsules will you give?

$$x \text{ cap} = 60 \text{ mg} \times \frac{1 \text{ gr}}{60 \text{ mg}} \times \frac{1 \text{ cap}}{\dfrac{1 \text{ gr}}{4}}$$

Simplify the complex fraction:

$$x \text{ cap} = 60 \text{ mg} \times \frac{1 \text{ gr}}{60 \text{ mg}} \times 1 \text{ cap} \times \frac{4}{1 \text{ gr}}$$

▶ **Answer:**   4 capsules

4. The order is to give 0.120 g of Seconal (secobarbital) suppository. On hand are suppositories containing gr i. How many suppositories will you give?

$$x \text{ supp} = 0.120 \text{ g} \times \frac{15 \text{ gr}}{1 \text{ g}} \times \frac{1 \text{ supp}}{1 \text{ gr}}$$

▶ **Answer:**   1.8 suppositories; therefore give 2

5. The physician ordered gr 1/64 of atropine sulfate. On hand are scored 2-mg tablets. How many tablets will you give?

$$x \text{ tab} = \frac{1 \text{ gr}}{64} \times \frac{60 \text{ mg}}{1 \text{ gr}} \times \frac{1 \text{ tab}}{2 \text{ mg}}$$

▶ **Answer:**   0.47 tablets; therefore, give 0.5, or 1/2, tablet

▲ MEDICATION FOR A COURSE OF THERAPY

Example 5.8 illustrates how to calculate the amount of medication needed to last a specified amount of time. In problems of this type, information is given concerning the number of doses per day and the amount of medication per dose.

When calculating medication for a course of therapy, the following are considered to be conversion factors:

1. How the medication is divided over 24 hours

    Example: q4h dose would give

    1 day = 6 doses

2. The amount of medication per dose

    Example: 500 mg PO would give

    1 dose = 500 mg

Example 5.8: The patient is to receive Gantrisin (sulfisoxazole) 1 g PO q.i.d. for 5 days. Tablets available are 0.25 g. How many tablets are needed to complete a 5 day course of therapy?

   The information provided in this problem includes:

Length of therapy	5 days
Number of doses per day	q.i.d. or 4 doses per day
Amount of each dose	1 gram per dose
Available medication	0.25 gram per tablet

Step 1: State the problem in equation form.

x tab = 5 days

Step 2: Identify the conversion factors needed to convert from days to tablets. The information needed from the problem to identify the conversion factors is: there are 4 doses per day; there is 1 gram per dose; there are 0.25 gram per tablet.

Three conversion factors are used:

A. Convert from days to doses.

   1 day = 4 doses

B. Convert from doses to grams.

   1 dose = 1 g

C. Convert from grams to tablets.

   0.25 g = 1 tab

Step 3: Put into the equation the form of each conversion factor that will cancel the unwanted labels and leave only the desired label on both sides of the equal sign.

$$x \text{ tab} = 5 \text{ days} \times \frac{4 \text{ doses}}{1 \text{ day}} \times \frac{1 \text{ g}}{1 \text{ dose}} \times \frac{1 \text{ tab}}{0.25 \text{ g}}$$

Step 4:   Cancel the labels that appear in both the numerator and the denominator on the same side of the equal sign.

$$x \text{ tab} = 5 \times \frac{4}{1} \times \frac{1}{1} \times \frac{1 \text{ tab}}{0.25}$$

Step 5:   Complete the required mathematical operations.

$$x \text{ tab} = 80 \text{ tab}$$

Therefore, 80 tablets are needed for 5 days of therapy.

Examples 5.9 and 5.10 illustrate how to calculate how long a given quantity of medication will last. The problems are worked in essentially the same manner as the previous example.

Example 5.9: The physician ordered 250 mg of Amoxil (amoxicillin) q8h PO. How many days will 300 ml of the medication last if each 5 ml contains 125 mg?

The information provided in this problem includes:

Total amount of medication	300 ml
Number of doses per day	q8h or 3 doses per day
Amount of each dose	250 mg per dose
Available medication	125 mg per 5 ml

Step 1:   State the problem in equation form.

$$x \text{ days} = 300 \text{ ml}$$

Step 2:   Identify the conversion factors needed to convert from milliliters to days. The information needed from the problem to identify the conversion factors is: there are 3 doses per day; there are 250 milligrams per dose; there are 125 milligrams per 5 milliliters.

Therefore, three conversion factors are used:

A. Convert from milliliters to milligrams.

$$5 \text{ ml} = 125 \text{ mg}$$

B. Convert from milligrams to doses.

$$250 \text{ mg} = 1 \text{ dose}$$

C. Convert from doses to days.

$$3 \text{ doses} = 1 \text{ day}$$

Step 3:   Put into the equation the form of the conversion factor that will cancel the unwanted labels and leave only the desired label on both sides of the equal sign.

$$x \text{ days} = 300 \text{ ml} \times \frac{125 \text{ mg}}{5 \text{ ml}} \times \frac{1 \text{ dose}}{250 \text{ mg}} \times \frac{1 \text{ day}}{3 \text{ doses}}$$

Step 4:   Cancel the labels that appear in both the numerator and the denominator on the same side of the equal sign.

$$x \text{ days} = 300 \times \frac{125}{5} \times \frac{1}{250} \times \frac{1 \text{ day}}{3}$$

Step 5: Complete the required mathematical operations.

x days $=$ 10 days

Therefore, 300 ml will last for 10 days.

Example 5.10: The order is for phenobarbital elixir gr 1/2 q12h. The concentration is 20 mg per 5 ml. How long will 150 ml last?

Step 1: State the problem in equation form.

x days $=$ 150 ml

Step 2: Identify the conversion factors needed to convert from milliliters to days. The information needed from the problem to identify the conversion factors is: there are 2 doses per day; there is 1/2 grain per dose; there are 20 milligrams per 5 milliliters.

A. Convert from milliliters to milligrams.

5 ml $=$ 20 mg

B. Convert from milligrams to grains.

60 mg $=$ 1 gr

C. Convert from grains to doses.

1/2 gr $=$ 1 dose

D. Convert from doses to days.

2 doses $=$ 1 day

Step 3: Put into the equation the form of each conversion factor that will cancel the unwanted labels and leave only the desired label on both sides of the equal sign.

$$x \text{ days} = 150 \text{ ml} \times \frac{20 \text{ mg}}{5 \text{ ml}} \times \frac{1 \text{ gr}}{60 \text{ mg}} \times \frac{1 \text{ dose}}{\dfrac{1 \text{ gr}}{2}} \times \frac{1 \text{ day}}{2 \text{ doses}}$$

Simplify the complex fraction.

$$x \text{ days} = 150 \text{ ml} \times \frac{20 \text{ mg}}{5 \text{ ml}} \times \frac{1 \text{ gr}}{60 \text{ mg}} \times 1 \text{ dose} \times \frac{2}{1 \text{ gr}} \times \frac{1 \text{ day}}{2 \text{ doses}}$$

Step 4: Cancel the labels that appear in both the numerator and the denominator on the same side of the equal sign.

$$x \text{ days} = 150 \times \frac{20}{5} \times \frac{1}{60} \times 1 \times \frac{2}{1} \times \frac{1 \text{ day}}{2}$$

Step 5: Complete the required mathematical operations.

x days $=$ 10 days

Therefore, 150 ml will last for 10 days.

▶ SOLVED PRACTICE PROBLEMS

1. The physician ordered 0.4 mg of atropine q6h. On hand are 1/300-gr tablets. How many tablets would be needed for 10 days of therapy?

$$x \text{ tab} = 10 \text{ days} \times \frac{4 \text{ doses}}{1 \text{ day}} \times \frac{0.4 \text{ mg}}{1 \text{ dose}} \times \frac{1 \text{ gr}}{60 \text{ mg}} \times \frac{1 \text{ tab}}{\dfrac{1 \text{ gr}}{300}}$$

Simplify the complex fraction.

$$x \text{ tab} = 10 \text{ days} \times \frac{4 \text{ doses}}{1 \text{ day}} \times \frac{0.4 \text{ mg}}{1 \text{ dose}} \times \frac{1 \text{ gr}}{60 \text{ mg}} \times 1 \text{ tab} \times \frac{300}{1 \text{ gr}}$$

▷ **Answer:** 80 tablets

2. The order is to give the patient 750 mg of Larodopa (levodopa) PO t.i.d. On hand are 0.25-g tablets. How many tablets would be needed for 10 days of therapy?

$$x \text{ tab} = 10 \text{ days} \times \frac{3 \text{ doses}}{1 \text{ day}} \times \frac{750 \text{ mg}}{1 \text{ dose}} \times \frac{1 \text{ g}}{1000 \text{ mg}} \times \frac{1 \text{ tab}}{0.25 \text{ g}}$$

▷ **Answer:** 90 tablets

3. The physician ordered gr XV of Tylenol (acetaminophen) elixir q6h. The label reads 120 mg per 5 cc. How many days will 600 cc of the medication last?

$$x \text{ days} = 600 \text{ cc} \times \frac{120 \text{ mg}}{5 \text{ cc}} \times \frac{1 \text{ gr}}{60 \text{ mg}} \times \frac{1 \text{ dose}}{15 \text{ gr}} \times \frac{1 \text{ day}}{4 \text{ doses}}$$

▷ **Answer:** 4 days

4. Phenobarbital gr i elixir is ordered q12h. The label states that 5 ml contains 20 mg. How many days will 300 ml last?

$$x \text{ days} = 300 \text{ ml} \times \frac{20 \text{ mg}}{5 \text{ ml}} \times \frac{1 \text{ gr}}{60 \text{ mg}} \times \frac{1 \text{ dose}}{1 \text{ gr}} \times \frac{1 \text{ day}}{2 \text{ doses}}$$

▷ **Answer:** 10 days

5. The order is for 150 mg of Amoxil (amoxicillin) q8h. How many days will 250 ml last if 5 ml of the medication contains 125 mg?

$$x \text{ days} = 250 \text{ ml} \times \frac{125 \text{ mg}}{5 \text{ ml}} \times \frac{1 \text{ dose}}{150 \text{ mg}} \times \frac{1 \text{ day}}{3 \text{ doses}}$$

▷ **Answer:** 14 days

CASE STUDIES

► Case Two

Mr. B., a 68-year-old male, was admitted with shortness of breath and severe edema of the lower extremities. His current diagnosis is congestive heart failure (CHF). Among his medical orders are the following: head of bed 45 degrees; oxygen at 4 L/min per nasal canula; restrict fluids to 1500 cc daily; 2-g sodium diet; digoxin elixir 125 μg PO q.d.; Lasix elixir 40 mg PO b.i.d.; Kay Ciel elixir 30 mEq PO b.i.d.

The ordered medications are labeled as follows:

Pharmacy Computer Printout Label

Name: Mr. B	**Room 124** **Date:** 07/07/xx
Order:	Kay Ciel Elixir 30mEq P.O., b.i.d.
Supplied:	20 mEq/15 cc
Directions:	Each tablespoon (15 cc supplying 20 mEq) should be diluted in 4 ounces of water or fruit juice.

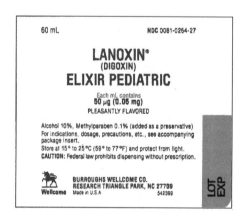

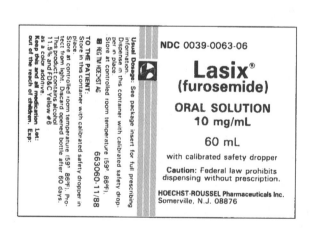

Refer to the medication labels to answer the following questions:

1. How many mcg of digoxin are in 1 cc of the elixir?
2. How many cc of digoxin will you administer?
3. How many times a day should the digoxin be given?
4. How many cc of Lasix would you give?

5. How many days will one bottle of Lasix last?
6. How many cc of Kay Ciel should you give?
7. How many ounces of fruit juice should be used to dilute 15 cc of Kay Ciel?
8. How many cc of fruit juice should you use to dilute 30 mEq of Kay Ciel?

For answers to the Case Study Two, see page 83.

► Case Three

M.C., a three-year-old child, is admitted with bacterial pneumonia. The child weighs 50 lb and has a history of seizures. The admit vital signs were temperature of 101.5F, pulse of 110, respiration rate of 25. The medication orders include 200 mg PO of Keflex (cephalexin) q6h and Dilantin (phenytoin) 50 mg PO q8h. The ordered medications are labeled as follows:

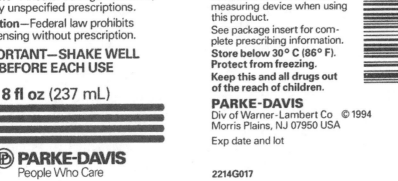

NDC 0777-2321-48 Ⓡ
100 mL (When Mixed) M-201

KEFLEX®
CEPHALEXIN FOR
ORAL SUSPENSION, USP

125 mg per 5 mL

◻DISTA

N 0071-2214-20

Dilantin-125®
(Phenytoin Oral Suspension, USP)

125 mg per 5 mL potency

Important—Another strength available; verify unspecified prescriptions.

Caution—Federal law prohibits dispensing without prescription.

IMPORTANT—SHAKE WELL BEFORE EACH USE

8 fl oz (237 mL)

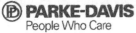

Ⓟ **PARKE-DAVIS**
People Who Care

6505-00-890-1110

THIS PRODUCT MUST BE SHAKEN WELL ESPECIALLY PRIOR TO INITIAL USE.

Each 5 mL contains phenytoin, 125 mg with a maximum alcohol content not greater than 0.6 percent.

Usual Dosage—Adults, 1 teaspoonful (5 mL) three times daily; children, see package insert.

Advice to Pharmacist and Patient—Patient must be advised to use an accurate measuring device when using this product.

See package insert for complete prescribing information.
Store below 30° C (86° F). Protect from freezing.
Keep this and all drugs out of the reach of children.

PARKE-DAVIS
Div of Warner-Lambert Co © 1994
Morris Plains, NJ 07950 USA

Exp date and lot

2214G017

(Used with permission of Bristol Laboratories, Division of Bristol-Meyers Squibb Company, Syracuse, New York 13221-4755)

Refer to the medication labels to answer the following questions.

1. How many mg of Keflex solution are in 5 cc of solution?
2. How many cc of Keflex will you administer?
3. How many times a day will Keflex be administered?
4. What is the manufacturer's maximum recommended dose of Keflex for this child in 24 hours?
5. What is the manufacturer's recommended maximum single dose of Keflex for this child?
6. Does the ordered dose of Keflex exceed the recommended single dose?
7. How many mg are in 5 cc of Dilantin suspension?
8. How many cc of Dilantin will you administer?
9. How many times a day will Dilantin be administered?

For answers to Case Study Three, see page 83.

► SELF-TEST

1. How many capsules of Tylenol (acetaminophen) would you administer if the physician ordered 600 mg for pain? On hand are 10 gr capsules.
2. The order is to give 1 oz of Maalox. How many tbsp would you give?
3. The physician ordered 2.0 g of neomycin. On hand are 500-mg tablets. How many tablets will you give?
4. How many tablets of codeine will you give if the physician ordered gr ss? On hand are 60-mg tablets.
5. How many ounces of Mylanta will you give if the physician orders 45 cc?
6. The order is to give 3 fl dr of Dimetapp (brompheniramine) elixir q4h PO. How many days will 360 cc of the medication last?
7. The physician orders gr 1/32 of Dilaudid (hydromorphone hydrochloride) q3–4h prn for pain. On hand are tablets gr 1/64 each. How many tablets will you give?
8. The order is for 15 fl dr of Kondremul. How many cc will you give?
9. The physician ordered erythromycin base 0.5 g q6h. On hand are 125 mg tablets. How many tablets will you give?
10. The order is to give 250 μg of Lanoxin (digoxin) q AM using 0.125 mg tablets. How many tablets will you give?
11. The order is to give chloral hydrate 1 g PO h.s. On hand are capsules containing $3\frac{3}{4}$ gr. How many capsules will you give?
12. The physician orders Fiorinal 30 mg. On hand are 1/8 gr capsules. How many capsules will you give?
13. The order is to give Achromycin (tetracycline) syrup 0.25 g PO q.i.d. The medication is available in syrup form, 125 mg per 5 cc. How many tsp will you give?
14. The physician ordered Synthroid (sodium levothyroxine) 25 μg q AM. Available are 0.05-mg tablets. How many tablets will you give?

Continued next page

▶ **Self-Test Continued**

15. The order is to give Keflex 500 mg q6h. The medication is supplied in a suspension, 5 cc containing 125 mg of medication. How many cc are needed for 14 days of therapy?

16. The physician ordered Slo-phyllin (theophylline) syrup 10 cc q8h. The medication is supplied 80 mg per 15 cc. How many mg of theophylline is the patient receiving per dose?

17. The order is to give 1/4 gr of Butisol (butabarbital) PO t.i.d. The medication on hand is 30 mg tablets. How many tablets will you give?

18. The physician's order is to give 300 μg of Catapres (clonidine) q8h. On hand are 0.1 mg tablets. How many tablets will you give?

19. The order is for 1 g of levodopa t.i.d. On hand are 250 mg tablets. How many tablets will you give?

20. The order is to give 0.750 g of Polycillin (ampicillin) oral suspension q.i.d. The medication is labeled 250 mg per 5 cc. How many tsp will you give?

For answers to the self-test, see below.

ANSWERS to Case Study Two

1. 50 μg/cc
2. 2.5 cc
3. One
4. 4 cc
5. 7.5 days
6. 23 cc
7. 4 oz
8. 180 cc

ANSWERS to Case Study Three

1. 125 mg
2. 8 cc
3. 4 times
4. 1136.4 mg
5. 284 mg
6. No, it does not exceed the recommended dose.
7. 125 mg
8. 2 cc
9. 3 times

ANSWERS to Self-test

1. 1 capsule
2. 2 tbsp
3. 4 tablets
4. 1/2 tablet
5. 1½ oz
6. 4 days
7. 2 tablets
8. 75 cc
9. 4 tablets
10. 2 tablets
11. 4 capsules
12. 4 capsules
13. 2 tsp
14. 1/2 tablet
15. 1120 cc
16. 53.33 mg
17. 1/2 tablet
18. 3 tablets
19. 4 tablets
20. 3 tsp

Parenteral Medications

6

Upon completion of Chapter 6, the student will be able to:

▸ Express the numerical value of the volume of medication to be administered in clinically feasible quantities given any syringe with any type of calibration.

▸ Correctly locate the appropriate calibration mark on a diagram of a U–100 insulin syringe for measuring the prescribed number of units of U–100 insulin.

▸ Correctly calculate, in milliliters, the volume of heparin needed to administer the prescribed dose given an appropriate concentration of heparin.

▸ Correctly calculate the volume of insulin needed, in milliliters, to administer the prescribed number of units with a T.B. syringe given any available concentration of insulin.

▸ Correctly calculate, in milliliters, the volume needed to administer the prescribed dose of any parenteral medication for injection.

▸ Correctly determine the amount of diluent needed to reconstitute a dry medication to produce an appropriate volume of medication to be given by the intramuscular or intravenous route.

▲ INTRODUCTION TO PARENTERAL MEDICATIONS

Parenteral medications are defined as those given by a route other than the gastrointestinal tract. In practice, parenteral refers to medications given by injection. Medications are administered by injection for local and systemic effects. Parenteral medication routes commonly used by nurses include intradermal, subcutaneous, intramuscular, and intravenous. The problems in Chapter 6 deal primarily with medications administered by the subcutaneous and intramuscular routes. Chapters 8–12 deal with calculations related to intravenous administration of fluids and medications.

Intradermal injections are used for skin-testing and tuberculin testing. Generally less than one milliliter of medication is given by the intradermal route using small-gauge, short needles.

Subcutaneous injections involve the administration of medication under the skin into the fat and connective tissue. Absorption of the medication is slow, and the drug action is prolonged. One to two milliliters can be given at one injection site using small-gauge, short needles. Sites commonly used include the arms, abdomen, back, and thighs.

Intramuscular injections are used to give a variety of medications directly into certain muscles. Medications given by this route act more rapidly than those given by subcutaneous injection. Up to 4 milliliters can be administered in one intramuscular injection site using medium-length, medium-to-large-gauge needles. Common sites for intramuscular injection include the following muscles: deltoid, dorsogluteal, ventrogluteal, and vastus lateralis.

Reading Syringe Calibrations

Intradermal and subcutaneous injections are normally administered using a 1 cc (ml) tuberculin (T.B.) syringe. Look at the T.B. syringe in Figure 6–1 and note that the syringe is calibrated on one side in ml (cc) and on the other side in minims. The members on the ml (cc) side of the 1 cc syringe indicate 0.1 cc calibrations. From one number to the next there are 10 smaller calibrations, which represent 0.01 cc increments.

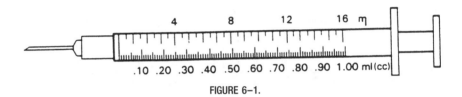

FIGURE 6–1.

Intramuscular injections are normally administered using a 3 cc or 5 cc syringe. Look at the 3 cc syringe in Figure 6–2 and note that this particular syringe is also calibrated on one side in ml (cc) and on the other side in minims. The numbers on the ml (cc) side of the 3 cc syringe indicate 0.5 cc calibrations. From one number to the next there are 5 smaller calibrations, which represent 0.1 cc increments.

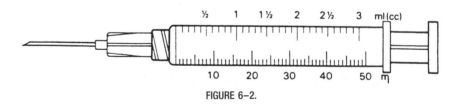

FIGURE 6–2.

Look at the 5 cc syringe in Figure 6–3 and note that this syringe, unlike those in Figures 6–1 and 6–2, is calibrated only in ml (cc). The numbers on the 5 cc syringe indicate 1 cc calibrations. From one number to the next there are 5 smaller calibrations, which represent 0.2 cc increments.

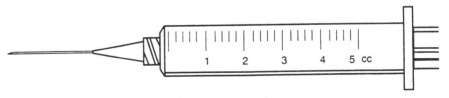

FIGURE 6–3. A 5-cc syringe.

▲ READING SYRINGE CALIBRATIONS

Answer the following questions using the syringes in Figure 6–4.

1. What are the smallest calibrations on syringe A?
2. What volume of medication is drawn up in syringe A?
3. Can syringe B be used to draw up 2.6 cc of medication?
4. What volume of medication is drawn up in syringe B?
5. Can syringe C be used to draw up 3.1 cc of medication?

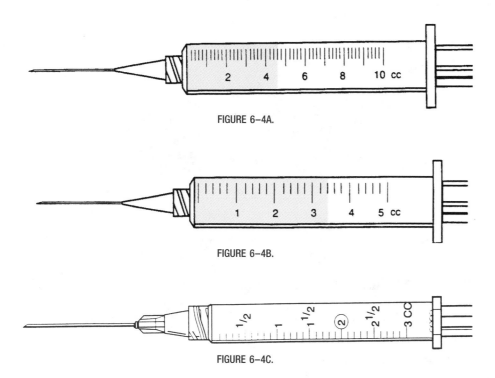

FIGURE 6–4A.

FIGURE 6–4B.

FIGURE 6–4C.

Sterile drug preparations given by injection are manufactured as solutions, suspension, and powders that require reconstitution before administration. Drug preparations are packaged in the following ways:

1. Single-dose vials: Closed glass containers with rubber stoppers; the medication is withdrawn by inserting a needle through the stopper
2. Multiple dose vials: Similar to single dose vials but contain more than one dose of medication
3. Ampules: Sealed glass containers; the top is broken to insert a needle to withdraw the medication
4. Prefilled syringes: Calibrated glass or plastic tubes with a needle attached

The volume of parenteral medication to be administered may be calculated in milliliters (cubic centimeters) or minims. However, since the manufacturer's medication concentrations are always expressed as amount of medication per milliliter (e.g., 50 mg per 1 ml), using minims is not necessary. In addition, answers calculated in milliliters will be more accurate.

▲ READING PARENTERAL MEDICATION DRUG LABELS

Medications Supplied as Solutions: Information regarding the concentration of a parenteral solution is printed on the drug label. Typically the label indicates routes by which the drug may be given. Refer to the Terramycin label in Figure 6–5.

    1. What is the concentration of Terramycin?
    2. What are the total number of milliliters (ml) in the vial?
    3. What are the total number of milligrams (mg) in the vial?
    4. What is the usual single adult daily dose?
    5. Is this a multidose vial?
    6. By which parenteral route may this Terramycin be given?

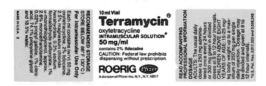

FIGURE 6–5.

Answers: 50 mg/ml; 10 ml; 500 mg; 250 mg; yes; IM only

Medications Supplied as Powders: Information regarding reconstitution of powdered forms of drugs may be found on the drug label or package insert. Refer to the information found in the package insert and the Keflin label in Figure 6–6.

    1. How many grams of Keflin are in the vial?
    2. How much diluent should be used to reconstitute each vial for IM injection?
    3. What is the concentration of the reconstituted solution?
    4. How many ml would you withdraw from the vial to give a 500 mg dose?

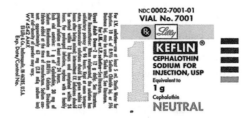

FIGURE 6–6.

DRUG INSERT INFORMATION: An IM injection of Keflin is prepared by adding 4 ml of sterile water for injection to each gram of Keflin. The resultant solution with 1 gram of Keflin has a total volume of 4.4 ml.

Answers: 1 g; 4 ml; 1 g/4.4 ml (or 227 mg/ml); 2.2 ml

► alert:

In drawing up parenteral medications, it is important to use an appropriately calibrated syringe to yield an accurate dose.

► critical decision point:

The order reads: *Give 35 units of regular human insulin SC now.* Generally available on your unit are 1 cc, 3 cc, and insulin syringes. (See Figure 6–7 and note the calibrations of the syringes.) You are ready to draw up the insulin but you do not have an insulin syringe. You look at the label on the Novolin insulin vial (see Figure 6–8) and determine that 0.35 ml of insulin contains 35 units. You find that you have available 1 cc and 3 cc syringes.

► decision/action:

You pick up the 3 cc syringe and note that the calibrations are in 0.1 ml increments. If you use this syringe you will have to estimate the 0.35 ml mark since the calibrations go from 0.3 ml to 0.4 ml on the syringe. You should NOT use this syringe since you will be unable to use it to measure the dose accurately. Your BEST choice is to use the 1 cc syringe to measure the required dose because it is calibrated in 0.01 ml increments and it allows you to measure a 0.35 ml quantity exactly.

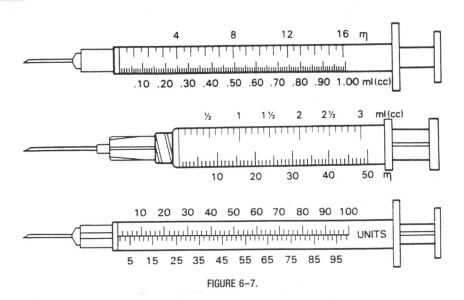

FIGURE 6–7.

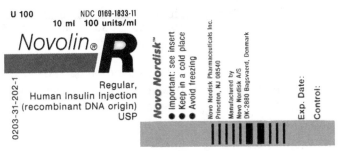

FIGURE 6–8.

▲ GENERAL PARENTERAL INJECTIONS

All calculations in this chapter on parenteral medications will be carried out using the dimensional analysis method of problem solving discussed in Chapter 2. There are no essential differences between calculations involving parenteral medications and those involving nonparenteral medications. The reader is referred to the first section of Chapter 5 for review.

Rounding answers. Answers to problems involving injection of parenteral medications measured in milliliters should be rounded to two decimal places if less than 1 milliliter, and rounded to one decimal place if greater than 1 milliliter. Answers calculated in minims or units (for insulin) should always be expressed in whole numbers only.

Examples 6.1–6.3 involve working with one or more conversion factors and include calculations with both simple and complex fractions.

Example 6.1: The order is to give Demerol (meperidine) 35 mg, IM q4h prn for pain. The medication is supplied in an ampule marked 50 mg per 1 cc. How much of the medication should you give?

Step 1: State the problem in equation form.

$$x \text{ cc} = 35 \text{ mg}$$

Step 2: Identify the conversion factor needed to convert from milligrams to cubic centimeters: 1 cc = 50 mg.

Step 3: Put into the equation the form of the conversion factor that will cancel the unwanted label (milligrams) and leave only the desired label (cubic centimeters) on both sides of the equal sign.

$$x \text{ cc} = 35 \text{ mg} \times \frac{1 \text{ cc}}{50 \text{ mg}}$$

Step 4: Cancel the labels that appear in both the numerator and the denominator on the same side of the equal sign.

$$x \text{ cc} = 35 \times \frac{1 \text{ cc}}{50}$$

Step 5: Complete the required mathematical operations.

$$x \text{ cc} = 0.7 \text{ cc}$$

Therefore, 0.7 cc will provide the ordered dose. (See Figure 6–9.)

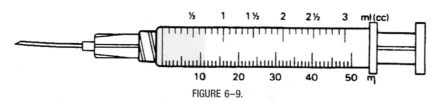

FIGURE 6–9.

Example 6.2: The order is to give 1/8 gr of morphine sulfate, IM q4h prn for pain. On hand are ampules labeled 10 mg per 1 cc. How much medication should you give?

Step 1: State the problem in equation form.

$$x \text{ cc} = \frac{1 \text{ gr}}{8}$$

Step 2: Identify the conversion factors needed to convert from grains to cubic centimeters. Two conversion factors are needed:

A. Convert from grains to milligrams.

1 gr = 60 mg

B. Convert from milligrams to cubic centimeters.

10 mg = 1 cc

Step 3: Put into the equation the form of each conversion factor that will cancel the unwanted labels (grains and milligrams) and leave only the desired label (cubic centimeters) on both sides of the equal sign.

$$x \text{ cc} = \frac{1 \text{ gr}}{8} \times \frac{60 \text{ mg}}{1 \text{ gr}} \times \frac{1 \text{ cc}}{10 \text{ mg}}$$

Step 4: Cancel the labels that appear in both the numerator and the denominator on the same side of the equal side.

$$x \text{ cc} = \frac{1}{8} \times \frac{60}{1} \times \frac{1 \text{ cc}}{10}$$

Step 5: Complete the required mathematical operations.

$$x \text{ cc} = 0.75 \text{ cc}$$

Therefore, 0.75 cc will provide the ordered dose. (See Figure 6–10.)

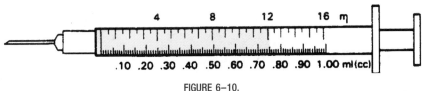

FIGURE 6–10.

Example 6.3: The order is to give 0.3 mg of atropine IM on call to surgery. The medication is provided in a vial labeled 1/150 gr per cc. How much should you give?

Step 1: State the problem in equation form.

$$x \text{ cc} = 0.3 \text{ mg}$$

Step 2: Identify the conversion factors needed to convert from milligrams to cubic centimeters. Two conversion factors are needed:

A. Convert from milligrams to grains.

60 mg = 1 gr

B. Convert from grains to cubic centimeters.

1/150 gr = 1 cc

Step 3: Put into the equation the form of each conversion factor that will cancel the unwanted labels and leave only the desired label on both sides of the equal sign.

$$x \text{ cc} = 0.3 \text{ mg} \times \frac{1 \text{ gr}}{60 \text{ mg}} \times \frac{1 \text{ cc}}{\dfrac{1 \text{ gr}}{150}}$$

The steps used to simplify the complex fraction are illustrated below:

A. $\dfrac{1 \text{ cc}}{\dfrac{1 \text{ gr}}{150}}$ is the same as: $1 \text{ cc} \div \dfrac{1 \text{ gr}}{150}$

B. Invert and multiply to get: $1 \text{ cc} \times \dfrac{150}{1 \text{ gr}}$

C. Substitute the simplified form of the expression into the equation in place of the complex fraction.

Therefore: $1 \text{ cc} \times \dfrac{150}{1 \text{ gr}}$ replaces $\dfrac{1 \text{ cc}}{\dfrac{1 \text{ gr}}{150}}$

$$x \text{ cc} = 0.3 \text{ mg} \times \frac{1 \text{ gr}}{60 \text{ mg}} \times 1 \text{ cc} \times \frac{150}{1 \text{ gr}}$$

Step 4: Cancel the labels that appear in both the numerator and the denominator on the same side of the equal sign.

$$x \text{ cc} = 0.3 \times \frac{1}{60} \times 1 \text{ cc} \times \frac{150}{1}$$

Step 5: Complete the required mathematical operations.

$$x \text{ cc} = 0.75 \text{ cc}$$

Therefore, 0.75 cc will provide the ordered dose.

► SOLVED PRACTICE PROBLEMS

1. The order is to give 60 mg of Garamycin (gentamicin) IM q8h. The vial is labeled 80 mg = 2 cc. How many cc should you give?

$$x \text{ cc} = 60 \text{ mg} \times \frac{2 \text{ cc}}{80 \text{ mg}}$$

► **Answer:** 1.5 cc

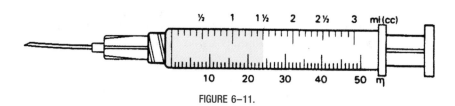

FIGURE 6–11.

2. The order is to give carbenicillin IM 800 mg q6h. The vial states that the concentration of the medication is 1 g per 2.5 cc. How many cc should you give?

$$x \text{ cc} = 800 \text{ mg} \times \frac{1 \text{ g}}{1000 \text{ mg}} \times \frac{2.5 \text{ cc}}{1 \text{ g}}$$

► **Answer:** 2 cc

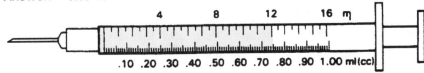

FIGURE 6-12.

3. The order is to give gr 1/8 of morphine sulfate IM q3–4h prn for pain. On hand is 1/6 gr per cc. How many should you give?

$$x \text{ cc} = \frac{1 \text{ gr}}{8} \times \frac{1 \text{ cc}}{\dfrac{1 \text{ gr}}{6}}$$

▶ **Answer:** 0.75 cc

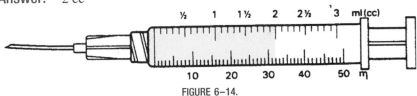

FIGURE 6-13.

4. The order is to give atropine 0.6 mg IM on call to surgery. On hand is an ampule labeled 1/200 gr per cc. How many cc should you give?

$$x \text{ cc} = 0.6 \text{ mg} \times \frac{1 \text{ gr}}{60 \text{ mg}} \times \frac{1 \text{ cc}}{\dfrac{1 \text{ gr}}{200}}$$

▶ **Answer:** 2 cc

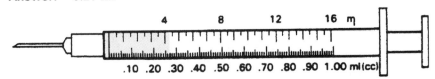

FIGURE 6-14.

5. The order is to give 4 mg of morphine stat. Available is 1/4 gr per ml. How many ml should you give?

$$x \text{ ml} = 4 \text{ mg} \times \frac{1 \text{ gr}}{60 \text{ mg}} \times \frac{1 \text{ ml}}{\dfrac{1 \text{ gr}}{4}}$$

▶ **Answer:** 0.27 ml

FIGURE 6-15.

▲ HEPARIN CALCULATIONS

Heparin is manufactured in different concentrations, which are expressed as a certain number of units of heparin per 1 cc. Commonly available concentrations of sodium heparin include: 5000 units per cc, 10,000 units per cc, 20,000 units per cc, and 40,000 units per cc. Heparin is administered subcutaneously or intravenously. It is recommended that a concentrated solution, usually 20,000 or 40,000 units per cc, be used for subcutaneous injection. For intermittent intravenous administration, less concentrated solutions, 5000 or 10,000 units per cc, are generally preferred.

Example 6.4: The physician ordered 10,000 units of heparin SC q12h. On hand are vials with 40,000 units per cc and 5000 units per cc. Which concentration should you use, and how much should you give?

Use 40,000 Units per cc

Step 1: State the problem in equation form.

$$x \text{ cc} = 10,000 \text{ U}$$

Step 2: Identify the conversion factor needed to convert from units to cubic centimeters: 1 cc = 40,000 U.

Step 3: Put into the equation the form of the conversion factor that will cancel the unwanted label and leave only the desired label on both sides of the equal sign.

$$x \text{ cc} = 10,000 \text{ U} \times \frac{1 \text{ cc}}{40,000 \text{ U}}$$

Step 4: Cancel the labels that appear in both the numerator and the denominator on the same side of the equal sign.

$$x \text{ cc} = 10,000 \times \frac{1 \text{ cc}}{40,000}$$

Step 5: Complete the required mathematical operations.

$$x \text{ cc} = 0.25 \text{ cc}$$

Therefore, 0.25 cc will provide the ordered dose. This dose is indicated on the 1-cc (T.B.) syringe illustrated in Figure 6–16.

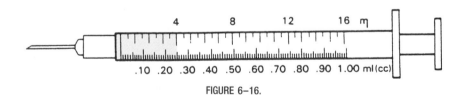

FIGURE 6–16.

Example 6.5: The order is to give Calciparine (heparin calcium) 11,000 units SC, q8h. Available is an ampule containing 12,500 units per 0.5 ml. How much medication should you administer?

Step 1: State the problem in equation form.

$$x \text{ ml} = 11,000 \text{ U}$$

Step 2: Identify the conversion factor needed to convert from units to ml: 0.5 ml = 12,500 U.

Step 3: Put into the equation the form of the conversion factor that will cancel the unwanted label and leave only the desired label on both sides of the equal sign.

$$x \text{ ml} = 11,000 \text{ U} \times \frac{0.5 \text{ ml}}{12,500 \text{ U}}$$

Step 4: Cancel the labels that appear in both the numerator and the denominator on the same side of the equal sign.

$$x \text{ ml} = 11,000 \times \frac{0.5 \text{ ml}}{12,500}$$

Step 5: Complete the required mathematical operations.

$$x \text{ ml} = 0.44 \text{ ml}$$

Therefore, 0.44 ml will provide the ordered dose. (See Figure 6–17.)

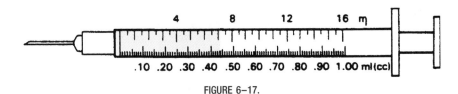

FIGURE 6–17.

▶ SOLVED PRACTICE PROBLEMS

1. How many cc of heparin will you administer if the physician orders 12,000 units q6h SC? Available is a vial containing 40,000 units per cc. How many cc should you give?

$$x \text{ cc} = 12,000 \text{ U} \times \frac{1 \text{ cc}}{40,000 \text{ U}}$$

▶ **Answer:** 0.30 cc

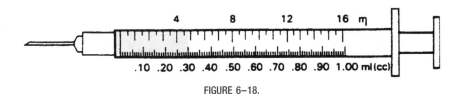

FIGURE 6–18.

2. How many minims of heparin will you administer if the physician orders 5000 units and available is 20,000 units per cc?

$$x \text{ m} = 5000 \text{ U} \times \frac{1 \text{ cc}}{20,000 \text{ U}} \times \frac{16 \text{ minims}}{1 \text{ cc}}$$

▶ **Answer:** 4 minims

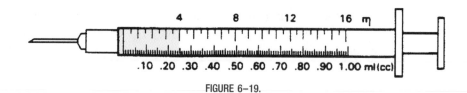

FIGURE 6–19.

3. The order is to give 14,500 units of heparin through the heparin lock q6h. On hand is a vial of 40,000 units per cc. How many cc should you use?

$$x \text{ cc} = 14,500 \text{ U} \times \frac{1 \text{ cc}}{40,000 \text{ U}}$$

► **Answer:** 0.36 cc

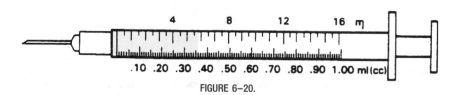

FIGURE 6–20.

4. The order is to give 9000 U of heparin SC q8h. Available are the following concentrations: 5000 units per cc and 20,000 units per cc. Which concentrations should be used? How many cc would you give?

$$x \text{ cc} = 9000 \text{ U} \times \frac{1 \text{ cc}}{20,000 \text{ U}}$$

► **Answer:** 0.45 cc of 20,000 units per cc

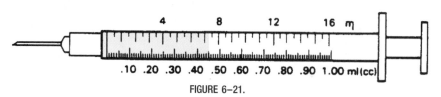

FIGURE 6–21.

5. The order is to give 18,000 units of Calciparine (heparin calcium) SC q8h. Available is a 0.8 ml ampule containing 20,000 units. How many cc would you give?

$$x \text{ cc} = 18,000 \text{ U} \times \frac{0.8 \text{ ml}}{20,000 \text{ U}}$$

► **Answer:** 0.72 cc

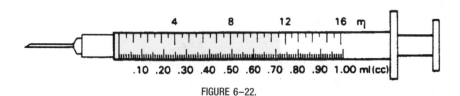

FIGURE 6–22.

▲ INSULIN CALCULATIONS

Insulin is available in three different concentrations: U–500, U–100, and U–40. The numbers, 500, 100, and 40, designate the units of insulin per 1 cc (Figure 6–23). Therefore, U–40 = 40 units per 1 cc, U–100 = 100 units per 1 cc, and U–500 = 500 units per 1 cc. Syringes are manufactured that are calibrated for the U–100 and U–40 insulin. If the concentration of the insulin ordered matches the calibration of the syringe used, no calculations are necessary since the syringes are marked in units.

U–100 insulin is the most commonly used concentration. U–500 insulin is ordinarily reserved for emergency situations or for mixing intravenous solutions. U–40 insulin is occasionally prescribed according to the preference of the physician.

Selecting insulin concentration. Since U–100 is the most widely used concentration, unless otherwise specified, all problems with insulin are calculated with U–100.

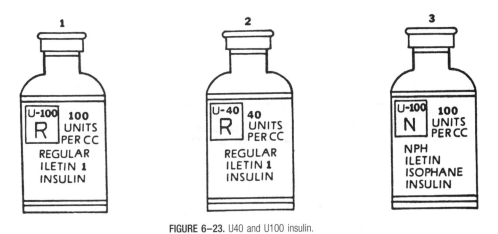

FIGURE 6–23. U40 and U100 insulin.

Example 6.6: The order is to give 30 units of Novolin 70/30 insulin each AM. Refer to the Novolin label in Figure 6–24. Using a 1-cc (T.B.) syringe, determine how much to give.

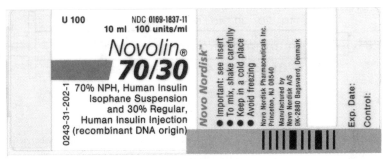

FIGURE 6–24.

Step 1: State the problem in equation form.

x cc = 30 U

Step 2: Identify the conversion factor needed to convert from units to cubic centimeter: 1 cc = 100 U.

Step 3: Put into the equation the form of the conversion factor that will cancel the unwanted label and leave only the desired label on both sides of the equal sign.

$$x \, cc = 30 \, U \times \frac{1 \, cc}{100 \, U}$$

Step 4: Cancel the labels that appear in both the numerator and the denominator on the same side of the equal sign.

$$x \, cc = 30 \times \frac{1 \, cc}{100}$$

Step 5: Complete the required mathematical operations.

$$x \, cc = 0.30 \, cc$$

Therefore, 0.30 cc is equal to 30 units of Novolin 70/30 insulin.

Note: It is recommended that you use cubic centimeters rather than minims when calculating insulin. This is needed to ensure the greatest possible accuracy of the dose.

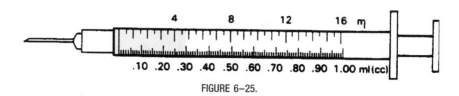

FIGURE 6–25.

Example 6.7: The order is to administer 18 units of regular insulin. Available are U–100 insulin and U–100 syringes. How much do you give?

Draw up the insulin to the 18 mark on the U–100 syringe. This dose is indicated on the U–100 syringe illustrated in Figure 6–26. No calculations are necessary.

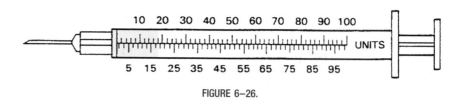

FIGURE 6–26.

Example 6.8: The order is to give 18 units of regular insulin as noted in Example 6.7 above. U–100 insulin is available but U–100 syringes are not. Using a 1 cc (T.B.) syringe, determine how much to give.

Step 1: State the problem in equation form.

$$x \, cc = 18 \, U$$

Step 2: Identify the conversion factor needed to convert from unit to cubic centimeters: 1 cc = 100 U.

Step 3: Put into the equation the form of the conversion factor that will cancel the unwanted label and leave only the desired label on both sides of the equal sign.

$$x\,\mathrm{cc} = 18\,\mathrm{U} \times \frac{1\,\mathrm{cc}}{100\,\mathrm{U}}$$

Step 4: Cancel the labels that appear in both the numerator and the denominator on the same side of the equal sign.

$$x\,\mathrm{cc} = 18 \times \frac{1\,\mathrm{cc}}{100}$$

Step 5: Complete the required mathematical operations.

$$x\,\mathrm{cc} = 0.18\,\mathrm{cc}$$

Therefore, 0.18 cc is equal to 18 units of U–100 insulin.

Note: When measuring U–100 insulin (100 units per 1 cc) in a 1-cc (T.B.) syringe, the number of units ordered will always equal an equivalent number of hundredths of a cubic centimeter. Therefore, to measure 18 units of U–100, measure to the 0.18 cc (18 hundredths) mark on the syringe. The 0.18 cc (18 hundredths) mark is illustrated on the 1-cc syringe in Figure 6–27.

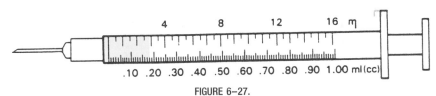

FIGURE 6–27.

Physicians frequently order both regular and NPH insulin to be given at the same time. These two insulins may be mixed in the same syringe. It is generally preferred to draw up the regular insulin first, then the NPH. This is illustrated in Example 6.9.

Example 6.9: The order is to administer 23 units of NPH and 12 units of regular insulin. Both types are available in U–100 strength. Using a U–100 insulin syringe, indicate the calibration marks on the syringe for each type of insulin. Both types of insulin may be drawn up in the same syringe.

First, draw up 12 units of regular insulin to the 12 mark. Second, draw up an additional 23 units of NPH insulin. This will bring the insulin in the syringe up to the 35 unit mark. This is indicated on the U–100 syringe illustrated in Figure 6–28.

Total insulin drawn = 12 units regular + 23 units NPH = 35 units.

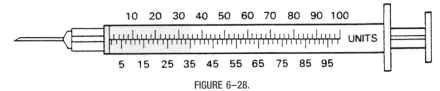

FIGURE 6–28.

It should be noted that in drawing up U–100 insulin or U–40 insulin it is always preferred to use the matching insulin syringe rather than a 1-cc (T.B.)

syringe. When it is necessary to use the 1-cc syringe, always use the cubic centimeter scale, even though the minim scale is calibrated on the syringe. This will ensure maximum accuracy in the dose given since multiplying by another factor (minims) will increase the margin of numerical error.

Example 6.10: The order is to give 80 units of regular insulin SC. Available is U–100 insulin but no corresponding U–100 syringes. Using a 1-cc (T.B.) syringe, calculate the dose required in cubic centimeters (cc).

Step 1: State the problem in equation form.

$$x \, cc = 80 \, U$$

Step 2: Identify the conversion factor needed to convert from units to cubic centimeters: 1 cc = 100 U.

Step 3: Put into the equation the form of the conversion factor that will cancel the unwanted label and leave only the desired label on both sides of the equal sign.

$$x \, cc = 80 \, U \times \frac{1 \, cc}{100 \, U}$$

Step 4: Cancel the labels that appear in both the numerator and the denominator on the same side of the equal sign.

$$x \, cc = 80 \times \frac{1 \, cc}{100}$$

Step 5: Complete the required mathematical operations.

$$x \, cc = 0.8 \, cc$$

Therefore, 0.8 cc equals 80 units. (See Figure 6–29.)

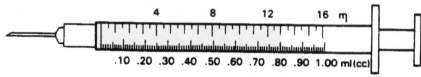

FIGURE 6–29.

Example 6.11: The physician ordered 10 units of U–40 regular insulin. Only U–100 is available. In an emergency, can the U–100 be used to administer the ordered dose?

U–100 can be used to administer the dose for the following reasons:

1. One unit is one unit (a set amount) regardless of the concentration of insulin in question (U–100 or U–40).
2. The *only* difference between 10 units of U–40 insulin and 10 units of U–100 insulin is the volume of solution in which it is dissolved. Since U–100 has 100 units per 1 cc and U–40 has only 40 units per 1 cc, it is clear that U–100 is more concentrated and would require a smaller volume to deliver the same amount (10 units) of insulin.
3. Therefore, 10 units of U–100 contains the same *amount* of insulin as 10 units of U–40, but in a smaller volume of solution.

▶ SOLVED PRACTICE PROBLEMS

1. How many cc of insulin, measured in a 1 cc (T.B.) syringe, will you give if the order is for 25 units of U–40?

$$x \, cc = 25 \, U \times \frac{1 \, cc}{40 \, U}$$

▶ **Answer:** 0.63 cc

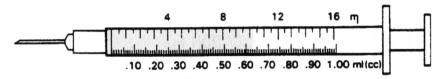

FIGURE 6–30.

2. How many cc of insulin, measured in a 1 cc (T.B.) syringe, will you give if the order is for 25 units of U–100 and there are no insulin syringes available?

$$x \, cc = 25 \, U \times \frac{1 \, cc}{100 \, U}$$

Recall that when measuring U–100 insulin (100 units per 1 cc) in a 1 cc syringe, the *number of units* ordered will always equal an equivalent number of *hundredths of a cubic centimeter*.

▶ **Answer:** 0.25 cc

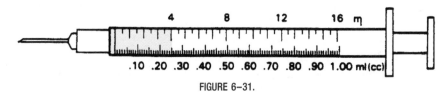

FIGURE 6–31.

3. The order is to give 10 units of U–40 insulin. Only U–100 insulin is available. How many cc of U–100 would contain the same amount of insulin as 10 units of U–40?

$$x \, cc = 10 \, U \times \frac{1 \, cc}{10 \, U}$$

Note that 10 units of insulin is the same regardless of what concentration it comes from. Only the volume needed to give the 10 units changes. Measured in cubic centimeters, 10 units of U–100 would be 0.10 cc while 10 units of U–40 is 0.25 cc. Both of these volumes contain the same amount (number of units) of insulin.

▶ **Answer:** 0.10 cc

4. The order is to give 18 units of regular insulin and 8 units of NPH insulin, both U–100. U–100 syringes are available for use. How would you draw up the medication?

Draw up the regular insulin to the 18 unit mark, then draw up 8 additional units of NPH insulin to the 26 unit mark. See Figure 6–32.

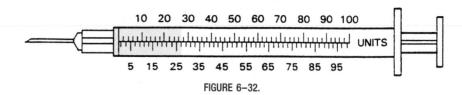

FIGURE 6–32.

▲ RECONSTITUTION OF MEDICATION FOR INJECTION

Medications that become unstable in solution over a period of time are often manufactured as dry powders. An appropriate diluent, such as sterile water or normal saline, must be added to these medications prior to administration. The process of adding the diluent is referred to as reconstitution of the medication. Most dry medications expand the volume of the diluent added to them. For example, when 23 cc of diluent are added to a dry vial of 5,000,000 units of penicillin G, the resulting volume is 25 cc.

Since many medications that are reconstituted are supplied in multiple-dose vials, directions for reconstitution must be strictly followed. Often a medication may be reconstituted with different amounts of diluent to produce various concentrations. In such cases, select a concentration that would provide the ordered dose in an appropriate volume for injection. Remember that it is generally recommended that no more than 3–4 ml be injected into one IM site. In some cases, however, it may be necessary to divide the dose and inject it into two separate sites.

Example 6.12: The physician's order is to give 2,500,000 units of penicillin G IM q6h. The medication is available in a 5,000,000 unit vial. How much of which concentration would you give?

Directions for reconstitution of the 5,000,000 unit vial indicate adding sterile water or isotonic sodium chloride as follows:

PENICILLIN CONCENTRATION	VOLUME OF DILUENT TO BE ADDED
250,000 units/ml	18 ml
500,000 units/ml	8 ml
1,000,000 units/ml	3 ml

The process of reconstitution of penicillin G is illustrated in Figure 6–33.

A concentration of 1,000,000 units/ml should be used. Using concentrations of 250,000 units/ml or 500,000 units/ml would result in volumes greater than 4 ml for IM injection of 2,500,000 units.

Step 1: State the problem in equation form.

$$x \text{ ml} = 2,500,000 \text{ U}$$

Step 2: Identify the conversion factor needed to convert from units to milliliters: 1 ml = 1,000,000 U.

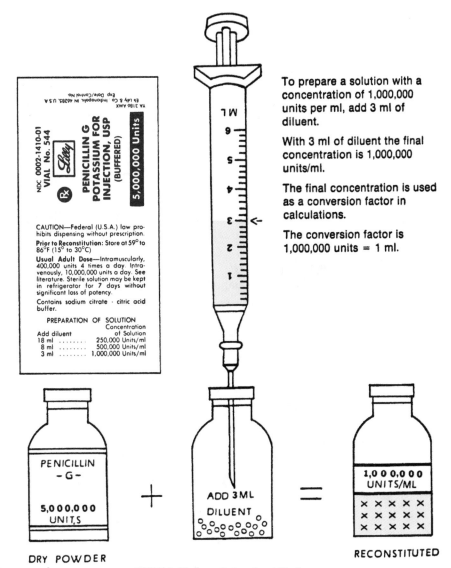

To prepare a solution with a concentration of 1,000,000 units per ml, add 3 ml of diluent.

With 3 ml of diluent the final concentration is 1,000,000 units/ml.

The final concentration is used as a conversion factor in calculations.

The conversion factor is 1,000,000 units = 1 ml.

FIGURE 6–33. Reconstitution of penicillin G.

Step 3: Put into the equation the form of the conversion factor that will cancel the unwanted label and leave only the desired label on both sides of the equal sign.

$$x \, \text{ml} = 2,500,000 \, \text{U} \times \frac{1 \, \text{ml}}{1,000,000 \, \text{U}}$$

Step 4: Cancel the labels that appear in both the numerator and the denominator on the same side of the equal sign.

$$x \, \text{ml} = 2,500,000 \times \frac{1 \, \text{ml}}{1,000,000}$$

Step 5: Complete the required mathematical operations.

$$x \, \text{ml} = 2.5 \, \text{ml}$$

Therefore, 2.5 ml will provide the ordered dose.

Example 6.13: The order is to give 300,000 units of penicillin G q4h IM. Directions for reconstitution on the 1,000,000 unit vial of powder indicate adding sterile water or isotonic sodium chloride to reconstitute. After reconstitution the following volumes and concentrations will be obtained:

PENICILLIN CONCENTRATION	VOLUME OF DILUENT TO BE ADDED	WITHDRAWABLE VOLUME
100,000 units per cc	9.6 cc	10 cc
200,000 units per cc	4.6 cc	5 cc
250,000 units per cc	3.6 cc	4 cc

For purposes of illustration, the volume needed to administer 300,000 units of medication with each of the above dilutions will be calculated.

Part 1: 9.6 cc of Diluent Added to Give 100,000 Units per cc

Step 1: State the problem in equation form.

$$x \text{ cc} = 300,000 \text{ U}$$

Step 2: Identify the conversion factor needed to convert from units to cubic centimeters: 1 cc = 100,000 U.

Step 3: Put into the equation the form of the conversion factor that will cancel the unwanted label and leave only the desired label on both sides of the equal sign.

$$x \text{ cc} = 300,000 \text{ U} \times \frac{1 \text{ cc}}{100,000 \text{ U}}$$

Step 4: Cancel the labels that appear in both the numerator and the denominator on the same side of the equal sign.

$$x \text{ cc} = 300,000 \times \frac{1 \text{ cc}}{100,000}$$

Step 5: Complete the required mathematical operations.

$$x \text{ cc} = 3 \text{ cc}$$

Part 2: 4.6 cc of Diluent Added to Give 200,000 Units per cc

Step 1: State the problem in equation form.

$$x \text{ cc} = 300,000 \text{ U}$$

Step 2: Identify the conversion factor needed to convert from units to cubic centimeters: 1 cc = 200,000 U.

Step 3: Put into the equation the form of the conversion factor that will cancel the unwanted label and leave only the desired label on both sides of the equal sign.

$$x \text{ cc} = 300,000 \text{ U} \times \frac{1 \text{ cc}}{200,000 \text{ U}}$$

Step 4: Cancel the labels that appear in both the numerator and the denominator on the same side of the equal sign.

$$x \text{ cc} = 300,000 \times \frac{1 \text{ cc}}{200,000}$$

Step 5: Complete the required mathematical operations.

$$x \text{ cc} = 1.5 \text{ cc}$$

Part 3: 3.6 cc of Diluent Added to Give 250,000 Units per cc

Step 1: State the problem in equation form.

$$x \text{ cc} = 300,000 \text{ U}$$

Step 2: Identify the conversion factor needed to convert from units to cubic centimeters: 1 cc = 250,000 U.

Step 3: Put into the equation the form of the conversion factor that will cancel the unwanted label and leave only the desired label on both sides of the equal sign.

$$x \text{ cc} = 300,000 \text{ U} \times \frac{1 \text{ cc}}{250,000 \text{ U}}$$

Step 4: Cancel the labels that appear in both the numerator and the denominator on the same side of the equal sign.

$$x \text{ cc} = 300,000 \times \frac{1 \text{ cc}}{250,000}$$

Step 5: Complete the required mathematical operations.

$$x \text{ cc} = 1.2 \text{ cc}$$

Therefore, to administer the ordered dose of 300,000 U of penicillin G administer *any* of the following:

3.0 cc of 100,000 U/cc
1.5 cc of 200,000 U/cc
1.2 cc of 250,000 U/cc

When using a multiple-dose vial, the dilution used, as well as the date of preparation, should be clearly marked for future use.

Example 6.14: The order is to give 1.5 g of Mefoxin (cefoxitin) IM q8h. Directions for reconstitution on the 2 g vial state:

MEFOXIN CONCENTRATION	AMOUNT OF DILUENT TO BE ADDED	WITHDRAWABLE VOLUME
400 mg/ml	4 ml for IM use	5.0 ml
180 mg/ml	10 ml for IV use	10.5 ml

Which dilution should be used and how many ml should be administered?

Use 4 ml of diluent since this is specified for IM use.

Step 1: State the problem in equation form.

$$x \text{ ml} = 1.5 \text{ g}$$

Step 2: Identify the conversion factor needed to convert grams to milliliters. Two conversion factors are needed:

A. Convert from grams to milligrams.

$$1 \text{ g} = 1000 \text{ mg}$$

B. Convert from milligrams to milliliters.

$$400 \text{ mg} = 1 \text{ ml}$$

Step 3: Put into the equation the form of each conversion factor that will cancel the unwanted labels and leave only the desired label on both sides of the equal sign.

$$x \text{ ml} = 1.5 \text{ g} \times \frac{1000 \text{ mg}}{1 \text{ g}} \times \frac{1 \text{ ml}}{400 \text{ mg}}$$

Step 4: Cancel the labels that appear in both the numerator and the denominator on the same side of the equal sign.

$$x \text{ ml} = 1.5 \times \frac{1000}{1} \times \frac{1 \text{ ml}}{400}$$

Step 5: Complete the required mathematical operations.

$$x \text{ ml} = 3.75 \text{ ml, which may be rounded to } 3.8 \text{ ml}$$

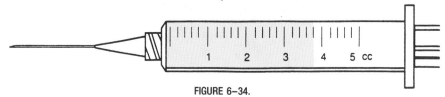

FIGURE 6–34.

► SOLVED PRACTICE PROBLEMS

1. The order is to give 350 mg of Prostaphlin (oxacillin) q4h IM. Directions for reconstitution of the 1 g vial state: Add 5.7 ml of sterile water. Each 1.5 ml will contain 250 mg of medication. How many ml will you give?

$$x \text{ ml} = 350 \text{ mg} \times \frac{1.5 \text{ ml}}{250 \text{ mg}}$$

► **Answer:** 2.1 ml

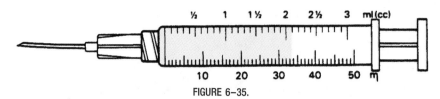

FIGURE 6–35.

2. The order is to give 1/4 g of Cefobid (cefoperazone) IM q12h. Directions for reconstitution of the 1 g vial state: Add 2.8 ml of sterile water to produce a concentration of 333 mg per ml. How many ml will you give?

$$x \text{ ml} = \frac{1 \text{ g}}{4} \times \frac{1000 \text{ mg}}{1 \text{ g}} \times \frac{1 \text{ ml}}{333 \text{ mg}}$$

► **Answer:** 0.75 ml

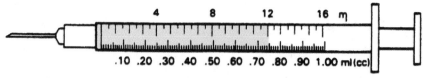

FIGURE 6–36.

3. The order is to give Pipracil (piperacillin) 750 mg IM q8h. Directions for reconstitution of the 2-g vial state: Add 4 ml of sodium chloride to produce a concentration of 1 g per 2.5 ml. How many cc will you give?

$$x \text{ cc} = 750 \text{ mg} \times \frac{1 \text{ g}}{1000 \text{ mg}} \times \frac{2.5 \text{ cc}}{1 \text{ g}}$$

▶ **Answer:** 1.9 cc

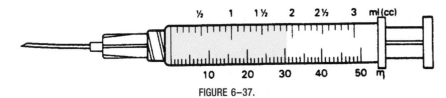

FIGURE 6–37.

4. The following refers to reconstitution of penicillin:

Diluent = Concentration
3.2 ml = 1,000,000 U/ml
8.2 ml = 500,000 U/ml
18.2 ml = 250,000 U/ml

Using the 3.2 ml diluent, how much penicillin must be used to administer 1.5 million units?

$$x \text{ ml} = 1,500,000 \text{ U} \times \frac{1 \text{ ml}}{1,000,000 \text{ U}}$$

▶ **Answer:** 1.5 ml

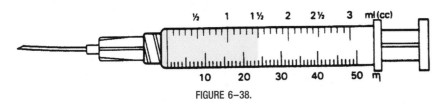

FIGURE 6–38.

5. The order is to give Polycillin-N (ampicillin) 700 mg IM q4h. The available medication is 1 g per vial. Directions for reconstitution state: Add 3.4 ml of recommended diluent to produce a withdrawable volume of 4 ml; the concentration will be 250 mg per ml. How many ml will you give?

$$x \text{ ml} = 700 \text{ mg} \times \frac{1 \text{ ml}}{250 \text{ mg}}$$

▶ **Answer:** 2.8 ml

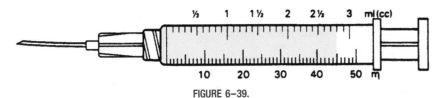

FIGURE 6–39.

CASE STUDIES

► Case Four

C.D., an 80-year-old obese female, has a history of deep vein thrombosis and is currently hospitalized with a diagnosis of acute urinary tract infection. During her hospitalization she developed left calf tenderness and was subsequently diagnosed as having thrombophlebitis of the left leg. The current medical orders for this patient include: bed rest; elevate left leg; Kefzol 250 mg IM q6h; sodium heparin 10,000 units SC q8h.

Penicillin G is sent from the pharmacy in a multiple-dose vial with the following label and insert information:

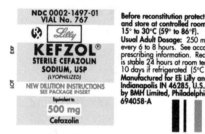

DOSAGE AND ADMINISTRATION

Kefzol may be administered intramuscularly or intravenously after reconstitution. Total daily dosages are the same for either route of administration.

Intramuscular Administration—Reconstitute as directed by Table 3 with 0.9% Sodium Chloride Injection, Sterile Water for Injection, or Bacteriostatic Water for Injection. Shake well until dissolved. Kefzol should be injected into a large muscle mass. Pain on injection is infrequent with Kefzol.

TABLE 3. DILUTION TABLE

Vial Size	Diluent to Be Added	Approximate Available Volume	Approximate Average Concentration
250 mg	2 mL	2 mL	125 mg/mL
500 mg	2 mL	2.2 mL	225 mg/mL
1 g*	2.5 mL	3 mL	330 mg/mL

*The 1-g vial should be reconstituted only with Sterile Water for Injection or Bacteriostatic Water for Injection.

FIGURE 6–40.

Refer to the medication label and package insert to answer the following questions:

The package insert included with the Kefzol (Figure 6–40) states: "Reconstitute as directed by Table 3 with 0.9% sodium chloride injection, sterile water for injection, or bacteriostatic water for injection."

1. How many mg of cefazolin sodium are contained in the vial?
2. What diluent(s) could be used?
3. If you add 2 ml of diluent, what is the resulting concentration of the reconstituted solution?
4. If you add 2 ml of diluent, how many ml should you administer?

Sodium heparin is available on the nursing unit in the following multiple-dose vials: 40,000 units per cc, 10,000 units per cc, 5000 units per cc.

5. Which is the most concentrated heparin solution?
6. Which concentration would allow you to administer the smallest volume of medication?
7. How many ml of which concentration will you give?

For answers to the Case Study Four, see page 111.

▶ Case Five

G.H., a 45-year-old female, is admitted with cellulitis of the lower left leg. Her admit temperature was 101F. The current medical orders include: bed rest, elevate left leg, Tazidime 250 mg IM q12h, and Nebcin (tobramycin) 60 mg IM q8h.

IM Tazidime and Nebcin are sent from the pharmacy in vials with the following labels:

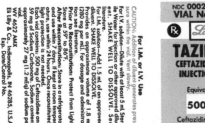
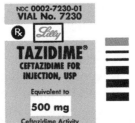

MANUFACTURER'S DRUG INFORMATION FOR TAZIDIME

For intramuscular administration, Tazidime should be reconstituted with 1 of the following diluents: Sterile Water for Injection, Bacteriostatic Water for Injection, or 0.5% or 1% Lidocaine Hydrochloride Injection.

	Amount of Diluent to be Added to the Vial (ml)	Approximate Available Volume (ml)	Approximate Concentration of Ceftazidime (mg/ml)
IM 500 mg Vial No7230	2.5	1.8	280
IM 1 gram Vial No7231	3.0	3.6	280

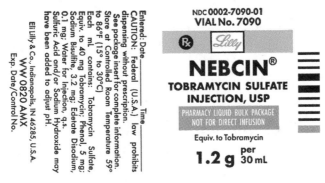

FIGURE 6–41.

Refer to the medication labels and answer the following questions.

1. How many mg of Tazidime are contained in the vial?
2. What diluent(s) may be used?
3. Following reconstitution, what is the concentration of Tazidime?
4. How many ml of Tazidime should you administer?
5. If refrigerated, how long may the reconstituted solution of Tazidime be stored?
6. How many mg of Nebcin are contained in each ml of solution?
7. How many cc of Nebcin equal the ordered dose of the drug?

For answers to the Case Study Five, see page 111.

► **SELF-TEST**

1. The order is to give gr 1/200 of atropine. On hand is an ampule labeled gr 1/150 per 2 ml. How many ml will you give?

2. The order is to give morphine sulfate IV push through a heparin lock. You are to give 6 mg and the available ampule is labeled 1/6 gr per ml. How many ml will you give?

3. The order is to give Vistaril (hydroxyzine hydrochloride) 75 mg q3–4h IM prn for nausea. The vial contains 100 mg per 2 cc. How many cc will you give?

4. The order is to give phenobarbital IM gr 1/4. On hand is a vial of 60 mg per cc. How many cc will you give?

5. The order is to give methicillin 0.6 g q12h. On hand is a vial labeled 150 mg per 1 ml. How many cc should you give?

6. The patient is to receive 12,000 units of sodium heparin q12h. On hand is a vial containing 40,000 units per cc. How many cc would you give?

7. The order is to give 5000 units of heparin SC q12h. Available are the following concentrations: 20,000 units per cc and 10,000 units per cc. How much of each concentration should you give?

8. The order is to give 5000 units of heparin SC. Using heparin, 10,000 units per ml, how many minims would you give?

9. The order is to give 7500 units of heparin SC q12h. On hand is a vial containing 40,000 units per cc. How many cc would you give?

10. The physician's order is to give 26 units of U–100 NPH insulin SC. Using a U–100 syringe, how would you measure the medication?

11. The order is to give 16 units of U–40 regular insulin SC. No U–40 syringes are available. How many cc would you give using a T.B. syringe?

12. The order is to give 20 units of U–100 regular insulin and 12 units of U–100 NPH insulin SC. Using a U–100 syringe, how would you measure the medication?

13. The physician ordered 24 units of U–40 regular insulin SC. How much U–100 would contain the *same amount* of insulin as 24 units of U–40?

14. The order is to give 20 units of U–100 regular insulin SC. No U–100 syringes are available. Using a T.B. syringe, how many cc will you give?

15. The order is to give 26 units of U–40 regular insulin SC. Using a U–40 syringe how would you measure the medication?

16. The physician has ordered Pipracil (pipercillin) IM 1.5 g q6h. The dilution table in the product information for a 4-g vial of Pipracil states: Add 7.8 ml of sterile water to the 4-g vial to produce a concentration of 1 g per 2.5 cc. How many cc will you give?

17. The order is to give 1 g of Mefoxin (cefoxitin) IM q8h. The directions for dilution on the 2 g vial state: Reconstitute with 4 ml of sterile water to give a withdrawable volume of 5 ml with an average concentration of 400 mg per ml. How many ml will you give?

Continued next page

> ▶ **Self-Test Continued**

18. The order is to give Omnipen (ampicillin) 350 mg q6h IM. The directions on the 250-mg vial state: Add 0.9 cc sterile water to produce a concentration of 125 mg per 0.5 cc. How many cc will you give?
19. The order is to give methicillin 0.75 g IM q4h. Directions on the 1 g vial state: Add 1.5 cc sterile water to produce 500 mg per cc. How many cc will you give?
20. The order is to give 1.25 g of Cefobid (cefoperazone) IM q12h. Directions on the 2 g vial state: Reconstitute with 5.6 ml of sterile water to give 333 mg per ml. How many ml will you give?

For answers to the self-test, see page 112.

1. 500 mg
2. Sterile water, 0.9% sodium chloride, bacteriostatic water
3. 225 mg/ml

4. 1.1 ml
5. 40,000 U/ml
6. 40,000 U/ml
7. 0.25 cc of 40,000 U/ml

1. 500 mg
2. Sterile water, bacteriostatic water, 0.5% or 1% Lidocaine Hydrochloride

3. 280 mg/ml
4. 89 ml
5. 7 days

ANSWERS to Case Study Four

ANSWERS to Case Study Five

ANSWERS to Self-test

1. 1.5 ml
2. 0.6 ml
3. 1.5 cc
4. 0.25 cc
5. 4 cc
6. 0.3 cc
7. 0.5 cc of 10,000 units per cc, or 0.25 cc of 20,000 units per cc
8. 8 m
9. 0.19 cc
10. Draw up the U–100 NPH to the 26 unit calibration mark on the syringe
11. 0.4 cc
12. Draw up U–100 regular insulin to the 20 unit calibration mark, and then draw up an additional 12 units of U–100 NPH in the same syringe to the 32 calibration mark.
13. 24 units of U–100 has the same amount of insulin (24 units), in a different volume, as does 24 units of U–40 insulin.
14. 0.2 cc
15. Draw up the U–40 insulin to the 26 unit calibration mark on the U–40 syringe.
16. 3.8 cc
17. 2.5 ml
18. 1.4 cc
19. 1.5 cc
20. 3.8 ml

Pediatric Medications Based on Body Weight

7

▲ OBJECTIVES

Upon completion of Chapter 7, the student will be able to:

- ► Apply the rules of problem solving by dimensional analysis to calculations involving medications based on body weight.

- ► Using the manufacturer's recommendation, correctly calculate the amount of medication needed to administer a single dose for a patient of any given weight.

- ► Using the manufacturer's recommendation, correctly calculate the amount of medication needed to equal the total daily dose for a patient of any given weight.

- ► Correctly calculate the minimum and maximum amounts of medication to administer based on the manufacturer's recommendations.

- ► Correctly determine if a prescribed dose of a medication exceeds the manufacturer's recommended dose given in grams, milligrams, or micrograms per kilogram per day or dose for a patient of any given weight.

▲ INTRODUCTION TO ADMINISTRATION OF PEDIATRIC MEDICATIONS BASED ON BODY WEIGHT

Under certain circumstances, medications are administered in doses based on the patient's body weight. This method is particularly useful when calculating drug doses for neonates, infants, and children. It provides reasonable medication doses since it is based on individual body size.

To avoid unreasonable dosage administration, pharmaceutical manufacturers provide specific information relevant to dosage and administration of each drug product. For most drugs, dosage information for adults and children is available. The information provided generally includes:

1. The single dose for an adult
2. Frequency of administration to an adult
3. Total amount of the drug to be administered to an adult in 24 hours
4. Single dose for a child, generally stated as milligrams per kilogram body weight per day
5. Frequency of administration to a child
6. Total amount of the drug to be administered to a child in 24 hours

Use of the milligrams per kilogram body weight per day (mg/kg/d) recommendation is commonly employed when calculating drug doses for children. When giving medications in this manner, adult doses are not exceeded, regardless of the weight of the child.

When medication dosage is prescribed on the basis of any single factor, such as body size, important clinical factors may be overlooked. These factors include the patient's general condition, concurrent drug therapy, available routes for drug administration, and the patient's individual response to drug therapy. Dosage information is based on current clinical practice and, as such, should be evaluated in accordance with each patient situation.

Using the manufacturer's recommendations, the nurse determines if a prescribed dose is a reasonable dose to administer. A reasonable dose does not exceed the manufacturer's recommendations for dosage as either a single dose or the total amount to be administered in 24 hours. The method of determining a reasonable dose based on the manufacturer's recommendation is described in this chapter.

Another method of determining doses appropriate to body size is based on body surface area. This method is frequently used in calculating doses of highly toxic drugs such as antineoplastic medications. Refer to Chapter 12 for information on calculating doses based on body surface area.

exercise

▲ READING PEDIATRIC MEDICATION LABELS

Recommended Pediatric Doses: Information regarding recommended pediatric doses may be printed directly on the drug label. As a general rule, the maximum child's dose will not exceed that maximum dose for an adult. Refer to the label in Figure 7–1.

1. What is the concentration of Vistaril?
2. What is the maximum daily adult dose?
3. What is the maximum daily pediatric dose for 6 yr and older?
4. What is the maximum daily pediatric dose for under 6 yr?

Vistaril®
(hydroxyzine pamoate)

ORAL SUSPENSION

*Each teaspoonful (5mL) contains
hydroxyzine pamoate equivalent
to 25 mg hydroxyzine hydrochloride.

USUAL DAILY DOSAGE
Adults: 1 to 4 teaspoonfuls 3-4 times daily
Children: 6 years and over–2 to 4 teaspoonfuls
daily in divided doses.
Under 6 years–2 teaspoonfuls daily
in divided doses.

**READ ACCOMPANYING
PROFESSIONAL INFORMATION.**

Store below 77°F (25°C)

Dispense in tight, light-resistant containers (USP)

**SHAKE VIGOROUSLY UNTIL PRODUCT IS
COMPLETELY RESUSPENDED.**

IMPORTANT: This closure is not child-resistant

DYE FREE FORMULA

CAUTION: Federal law
prohibits dispensing
without prescription.

05-0844-00-4
MADE IN USA
4387

NDC 0069-5440-93

1 Pint (473 mL)

Vistaril®
(hydroxyzine pamoate)

ORAL SUSPENSION

E005A
EXP 1 MAY 00

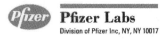
25 mg/5 mL*

For Oral Use Only

3 0069-5440-93 9

Pfizer **Pfizer Labs**
Division of Pfizer Inc, NY, NY 10017

FIGURE 7–1.

Answers: 25 mg/5 ml; 16 tsp; 4 tsp; 2 tsp

Maximum Recommended Pediatric Doses: Dosage information on a drug label may be given in terms mg/kg/d. Additional information may be found in drug information literature. Both sources of information should be used to determine the maximum daily dose allowed for a child. Refer to the label in Figure 7–2.

1. What is the concentration of reconstituted Ceclor?
2. How much water must be added to reconstitute Ceclor?
3. What is the usual daily dose for an adult?
4. What is the usual daily dose for a child?
5. What is the daily dose for a child with otitis media?

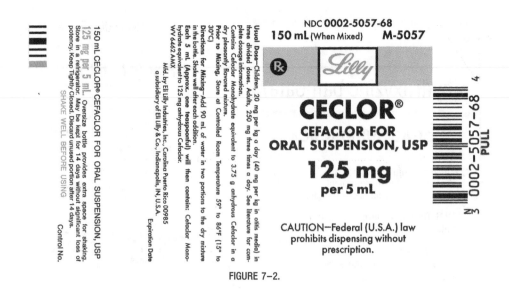

FIGURE 7-2.

Answers: 125 mg/5 ml; 45 ml; 750 mg; 20 mg/kg/d; 40 mg/kg/d

► alert:

It is necessary to determine the maximum permissible daily dose of a medication for a child and ensure that this dose is not exceeded.

► critical decision point:

The order reads: *Give 400 mg of cefaclor PO q8h.* The patient, who weighs 22 kg, has otitis media. You check the drug label (Figure 7–2) and note that normal adult dose is 250 mg q8h and that the recommended dose for a child with otitis media is 40 mg/kg/d. You look up the drug in the ***Nurses Drug Guide*** and find that the maximum adult dose is 500 mg q8h (1500 mg/day) and that the child's dose should not exceed 1 g/d. The current order requires 400 mg every 8 hours or a total daily dose of 1200 mg.

► decision/action:

Based on the recommendation of 40 mg/kg/d, you calculate that a 22-kg child should receive 880 mg daily. This dose of 400 mg q8h *does exceed* both the maximum recommended dose for this child and the general maximum for children, which is 1 g/day. The medication should be held and the order clarified.

▲ CALCULATING PEDIATRIC DOSAGE BASED ON BODY WEIGHT

In problems of this type, the question asked is how much medication is recommended for a pediatric patient of a particular weight for a *single dose* or for a *total daily dose*. To determine the amount of medication to give, the beginning part of the problem is put into one of the following forms:

Medication for a Single Dose

$$\frac{? \, mg}{wt \times dose} = \text{How many milligrams should be given to a patient of a particular } \textit{weight} \text{ for a } \textit{single dose?}$$

Medication for a Total Daily Dose

$$\frac{? \, mg}{wt \times day} = \text{How many milligrams should be given to a patient of a particular } \textit{weight} \text{ for a } \textit{total daily dose?}$$

It is important to include the term (wt × dose) or (wt × day) in the denominator since the number of milligrams calculated depends both on the patient's weight and whether a single or total daily dose is being determined.

As in previous chapters, calculations of pediatric medications based on body weight are carried out using the dimensional analysis method of problem solving discussed in Chapter 2. The application of the method to pediatric dosages based on body weight is illustrated in Example 7.1.

Rounding answers. Precision with pediatric dosage calculations is extremely important. The following are suggestions for rounding answers in a consistent fashion: When calculating manufacturer's recommended doses, medication weights less than 1 milligram should be rounded to two decimal places. Weights between 1 milligram and 10 milligrams may be rounded to one decimal place, while weights greater than 10 milligrams may be rounded to whole numbers. Medication volumes less than 1 milliliter should be rounded to two decimal places, while volumes greater than 1 milliliter may be rounded to one decimal place.

Example 7.1: The recommended dose of phenobarbital is 5 mg kg per day (5 mg/kg/d) in 2 equally divided doses. For an infant weighing 10 kg, how many mg per dose, given b.i.d., are recommended?

▶ Rules of Problem Solving by Dimensional Analysis

 One side of an equation can be multiplied by an appropriate conversion factor without changing the value of the equation.

◀ RULE 1

▶ Application of Rule 1

When calculating medication dosages based on body weight, the following are considered to be conversion factors:

1. How the medication is divided over a 24-hour period

   In the problem given, the conversion factor is 1 day = 2 doses. This conversion factor can be put into the problem in either of two forms:

   $$\frac{1 \, day}{2 \, doses} \quad \text{or} \quad \frac{2 \, doses}{1 \, day}$$

2. The particular weight of the pediatric patient

In the problem given, the conversion factor is 10 kg = weight. This conversion factor can be put into the problem in either of two forms:

$$\frac{10 \text{ kg}}{\text{wt}} \quad \text{or} \quad \frac{\text{wt}}{10 \text{ kg}}$$

RULE 2 ▶

 The problem is correctly set up when all labels cancel from both the numerator and the denominator except the labels that are desired in the answer.

▶ Application of Rule 2

1. In the problem given, the following question is asked: How many milligrams are recommended for an infant of this particular weight for a *single dose* in order to provide 5 mg per kg per day in two equal doses?

2. Stated in an equation form, the problem is

$$\frac{x \text{ mg}}{\text{wt} \times \text{dose}} = \frac{5 \text{ mg}}{\text{kg} \times \text{day}} \text{ (in 2 equal doses)}$$

Since the dose (5 mg) is determined by weight (kg) and time frame (day).

Note: The first term to the right of the equal sign is the manufacturer's recommended dose since this is what determines the amount of medication that should be ordered.

$$\frac{x \text{ mg}}{\text{wt} \times \text{dose}} = \frac{5 \text{ mg}}{\text{kg} \times \text{day}} \quad \begin{array}{l} \text{To solve the problem, convert kg to wt} \\ \text{and day to dose.} \end{array}$$

3. The conversion factors, 10 kg = wt and 1 day = 2 doses, are put into the equation as fractions. The form of each fraction used is that which will cancel the unwanted labels (kilograms and day) and leave only the desired labels (milligrams per weight per dose) on both sides of the equal sign.

$$\frac{x \text{ mg}}{\text{wt} \times \text{dose}} = \frac{5 \text{ mg}}{\text{kg} \times \text{day}} \times \frac{10 \text{ kg}}{\text{wt}} \times \frac{1 \text{ day}}{2 \text{ doses}}$$

The equation can now be read: *x* milligrams per given weight per dose equal 5 milligrams per kilogram per day when it is true that 10 kilograms is the given weight, and when it is true that in 1 day there are 2 doses.

4. Cancel labels that appear in both the numerator and denominator on the same side of the equal sign.

$$\frac{x \text{ mg}}{\text{wt} \times \text{dose}} = 5 \text{ mg} \times \frac{10}{\text{wt}} \times \frac{1}{2 \text{ doses}}$$

5. Completing the required mathematical operations gives:

$$\frac{x \text{ mg}}{\text{wt} \times \text{dose}} = \frac{5 \text{ mg} \times 10 \times 1}{\text{wt} \times 2 \text{ doses}} = \frac{25 \text{ mg}}{\text{wt} \times \text{dose}}$$

Therefore, 25 mg will provide the recommended dose for a 10 kg infant.

The method of problem solving by dimensional analysis illustrated will be used throughout this chapter. For simplicity the method will be reduced to the same five-step procedure used in previous chapters.

▲ CALCULATING SINGLE PEDIATRIC DOSES

Example 7.2: The recommendation for pediatric Tylenol (acetaminophen) is 25 mg/kg/d in 4 equally divided doses. How many mg are recommended for each dose for a 15-kg child?

Step 1: State the problem in equation form.

$$\frac{x \text{ mg}}{\text{wt} \times \text{dose}} = \frac{25 \text{ mg}}{\text{kg} \times \text{day}} \text{ (in 4 equal doses)}$$

Step 2: Identify the conversion factors needed to convert from mg/kg/d to mg/wt/dose. The information needed from the problem to identify the conversion factors is: The patient weighs 15 kg; and there are 4 doses per day.

Two conversion factors are used:

A. Convert from kilograms to weight.

15 kg = wt

B. Convert from day to dose.

1 day = 4 doses

Step 3: Put into the equation the form of each conversion factor that will cancel the unwanted labels (kilograms and day) and leave only the desired labels (milligrams per weight per dose) on both sides of the equal sign.

$$\frac{x \text{ mg}}{\text{wt} \times \text{dose}} = \frac{25 \text{ mg}}{\text{kg} \times \text{day}} \times \frac{15 \text{ kg}}{\text{wt}} \times \frac{1 \text{ day}}{4 \text{ doses}}$$

Step 4: Cancel the labels that appear in both the numerator and the denominator on the same side of the equal sign.

$$\frac{x \text{ mg}}{\text{wt} \times \text{dose}} = 25 \text{ mg} \times \frac{15}{\text{wt}} \times \frac{1}{4 \text{ doses}}$$

Step 5: Complete the required mathematical operations.

$$\frac{x \text{ mg}}{\text{wt} \times \text{dose}} = \frac{93.75 \text{ mg}}{\text{wt} \times \text{dose}}$$

Therefore, 94 mg will provide the recommended dose for a 15-kg child.

Example 7.3: The recommendation for preoperative atropine is 0.02 mg/kg/dose. The infant weighs 12 kg. The atropine is supplied 0.1 mg per cc. How many cc are recommended for a single dose?

Step 1: State the problem in equation form.

$$\frac{x \text{ cc}}{\text{wt} \times \text{dose}} = \frac{0.02 \text{ mg}}{\text{kg} \times \text{dose}}$$

Step 2: Identify the conversion factors needed to convert from mg/kg/dose to cc/wt/dose. The information needed from the problem to identify the conversion factors is: the patient weighs 12 kg; and there is 0.1 mg of atropine per cc.

Two conversion factors are used:

A. Convert from kilograms to weight.

  12 kg = wt

B. Convert from milligrams to cubic centimeters.

  0.1 mg = 1 cc

Step 3: Put into the equation the form of each conversion factor that will cancel the unwanted labels and leave only the desired labels on both sides of the equal sign.

$$\frac{x \text{ cc}}{\text{wt} \times \text{dose}} = \frac{0.02 \text{ mg}}{\text{kg} \times \text{dose}} \times \frac{12 \text{ kg}}{\text{wt}} \times \frac{1 \text{ cc}}{0.1 \text{ mg}}$$

Step 4: Cancel the labels that appear in both the numerator and the denominator on the same side of the equal sign.

$$\frac{x \text{ cc}}{\text{wt} \times \text{dose}} = \frac{0.02}{\text{dose}} \times \frac{12}{\text{wt}} \times \frac{1 \text{ cc}}{0.1}$$

Step 5: Complete the required mathematical operations.

$$\frac{x \text{ cc}}{\text{wt} \times \text{dose}} = \frac{2.4 \text{ cc}}{\text{dose} \times \text{wt}}$$

Therefore, 2.4 cc will provide the recommended dose for a 12 kg infant.

Example 7.4: The recommendation is tetracycline 40 mg/kg/d in equal doses divided q6h. The child weighs 67.5 lb. How many mg are recommended for each dose?

Step 1: State the problem in equation form.

$$\frac{x \text{ mg}}{\text{wt} \times \text{dose}} = \frac{40 \text{ mg}}{\text{kg} \times \text{day}} \text{ (in 4 equal doses)}$$

Step 2: Identify the conversion factors needed to convert from mg/kg/d to mg/wt/dose. The information needed from the problem to identify the conversion factors is: The patient weighs 67.5 lb; and there are 4 doses per day.

Three conversion factors are used:

A. Convert from kilograms to pounds.

  1 kg = 2.2 lb

B. Convert from pounds to weight.

67.5 lb = wt

C. Convert from day to doses.

1 day = 4 doses

Step 3: Put into the equation the form of each conversion factor that will cancel the unwanted labels and leave only the desired labels on both sides of the equal sign.

$$\frac{x \text{ mg}}{\text{wt} \times \text{dose}} = \frac{40 \text{ mg}}{\text{kg} \times \text{day}} \times \frac{1 \text{ kg}}{2.2 \text{ lb}} \times \frac{67.5 \text{ lb}}{\text{wt}} \times \frac{1 \text{ day}}{4 \text{ doses}}$$

Step 4: Cancel the labels that appear in both the numerator and the denominator on the same side of the equal sign.

$$\frac{x \text{ mg}}{\text{wt} \times \text{dose}} = 40 \text{ mg} \times \frac{1}{2.2} \times \frac{67.5}{\text{wt}} \times \frac{1}{4 \text{ doses}}$$

Step 5: Complete the required mathematical operations.

$$\frac{x \text{ mg}}{\text{wt} \times \text{dose}} = \frac{306.8 \text{ mg}}{\text{wt} \times \text{dose}}$$

Therefore, 307 mg will provide the recommended dose for a 67.5 lb child.

▶ SOLVED PRACTICE PROBLEMS

1. The recommended dose of Diuril (chlorothiazide) is 25 mg/kg/day in 3 equally divided doses. The infant weighs 6 kg. Determine the recommended number of mg per dose.

$$\frac{x \text{ mg}}{\text{wt} \times \text{dose}} = \frac{25 \text{ mg}}{\text{kg} \times \text{day}} \times \frac{6 \text{ kg}}{\text{wt}} \times \frac{1 \text{ day}}{3 \text{ doses}}$$

▷ **Answer:** 50 mg

2. The recommended dose of aspirin is 65 mg/kg/day divided equally q6h. The child weighs 18.4 kg. Determine the recommended number of mg per dose.

$$\frac{x \text{ mg}}{\text{wt} \times \text{dose}} = \frac{65 \text{ mg}}{\text{kg} \times \text{day}} \times \frac{18.4 \text{ kg}}{\text{wt}} \times \frac{1 \text{ day}}{4 \text{ doses}}$$

▷ **Answer:** 299 mg

3. The recommendation is Atarax (hydroxyzine) 2 mg/kg/day in 3 equally divided doses. The child weighs 60 lb. Determine the recommended number of mg per dose.

$$\frac{x \text{ mg}}{\text{wt} \times \text{dose}} = \frac{2 \text{ mg}}{\text{kg} \times \text{day}} \times \frac{1 \text{ kg}}{2.2 \text{ lb}} \times \frac{60 \text{ lb}}{\text{wt}} \times \frac{1 \text{ day}}{3 \text{ doses}}$$

▷ **Answer:** 18 mg

4. The recommendation is phenobarbital 6 mg/kg/24 h to be given in 3 equally divided doses. The medication is supplied in liquid form, 7.5 mg per 5 cc. The infant weighs 9 kg. Determine the recommended number of cc per dose.

$$\frac{x \text{ cc}}{\text{wt} \times \text{dose}} = \frac{6 \text{ mg}}{\text{kg} \times \text{day}} \times \frac{9 \text{ kg}}{\text{wt}} \times \frac{1 \text{ day}}{3 \text{ doses}} \times \frac{5 \text{ cc}}{7.5 \text{ mg}}$$

▶ **Answer:** 12 cc

5. The recommendation is gentamicin 6 mg/kg/day in equal doses divided q8h. The medication is available in multiple dose vials of 20 mg per 2 cc. How many cc would be recommended for an infant weighing 11 lb, 4 oz?

$$\frac{x \text{ cc}}{\text{wt} \times \text{dose}} = \frac{6 \text{ mg}}{\text{kg} \times \text{day}} \times \frac{1 \text{ kg}}{2.2 \text{ lb}} \times \frac{11.25 \text{ lb}}{\text{wt}} \times \frac{1 \text{ day}}{3 \text{ doses}} \times \frac{2 \text{ cc}}{20 \text{ mg}}$$

▶ **Answer:** 1 cc

▲ CALCULATING TOTAL DAILY PEDIATRIC DOSES

Calculation of a total daily dose is similar to calculation of a single dose. In the case of the total daily dose, the problem is solved to determine the amount of medication per given weight per day rather than per dose.

Example 7.5: The recommended dose of erythromycin is 10 mg/kg t.i.d. The child weighs 23 lb, 6 oz. Determine the recommended total daily dose.

Note: The recommendation is stated in terms of a *single dose.* 10 mg/kg t.i.d. means 10 mg per kg per *dose* (given three times a day) and *not* 10 mg per kg per *day* (divided in three doses).

Step 1: State the problem in equation form.

$$\frac{x \text{ mg}}{\text{wt} \times \text{day}} = \frac{10 \text{ mg}}{\text{kg} \times \text{dose}}$$

Step 2: Identify the conversion factors needed to convert from mg/kg/dose to mg/wt/d. The information needed from the problem to identify the conversion factors is: The patient weighs 23 lb, 6 oz (23.38 lb); and there are 3 doses per day.

Three conversion factors are used:

A. Convert from kilograms to pounds.

1 kg = 2.2 lb

B. Convert from pounds to weight.

23 lb, 6 oz (23.38 lb) = wt

C. Convert from dose to day.

3 doses = 1 day

Step 3: Put into the equation the form of each conversion factor that will cancel the unwanted labels and leave only the desired labels on both sides of the equal sign.

$$\frac{x \text{ mg}}{\text{wt} \times \text{day}} = \frac{10 \text{ mg}}{\text{kg} \times \text{dose}} \times \frac{1 \text{ kg}}{2.2 \text{ lb}} \times \frac{23.38 \text{ lb}}{\text{wt}} \times \frac{3 \text{ doses}}{1 \text{ day}}$$

Step 4: Cancel the labels that appear in both the numerator and the denominator on the same side of the equal sign.

$$\frac{x \text{ mg}}{\text{wt} \times \text{day}} = 10 \text{ mg} \times \frac{1}{2.2} \times \frac{23.38}{\text{wt}} \times \frac{3}{1 \text{ day}}$$

Step 5: Complete the required mathematical operations.

$$\frac{x \text{ mg}}{\text{wt} \times \text{day}} = \frac{318.8 \text{ mg}}{\text{day} \times \text{wt}}$$

Therefore, the recommended daily dose is 319 mg for a 23.38-lb child.

Example 7.6: The recommended neonatal digitalizing dose of digoxin is 50 μg/kg given in three doses, 8 hours apart and divided 1/2 total dose, 1/4 total dose, 1/4 total dose. Determine the *total daily dose* and also each of *three* q8h *doses* for a newborn weighing 1500 g.

Note: The medication is given in 3 doses in a 24-hour period, but the doses are not equally divided. Therefore, it is necessary to calculate the total dose and from that determine the three doses (1/2, 1/4, and 1/4).

Step 1: State the equation needed to find the total daily dose.

$$\frac{x \mu\text{g}}{\text{wt} \times \text{day}} = \frac{50 \mu\text{g}}{\text{kg} \times \text{day}}$$

Step 2: Identify the conversion factors needed to convert from μg/kg/d to μg/wt/d. The information needed from the problem to identify the conversion factors is: wt = 1500 g.

Two conversion factors are used:

A. Convert from kilograms to grams.

   1 kg = 1000 g

B. Convert from grams to weight.

   1500 g = wt

Step 3: Put into the equation the form of each conversion factor that will cancel the unwanted labels and leave only the desired labels on both sides of the equal sign.

$$\frac{x \mu\text{g}}{\text{wt} \times \text{day}} = \frac{50 \mu\text{g}}{\text{kg} \times \text{day}} \times \frac{1 \text{ kg}}{1000 \text{ g}} \times \frac{1500 \text{ g}}{\text{wt}}$$

Step 4: Cancel the labels that appear in both the numerator and the denominator on the same side of the equal sign.

$$\frac{x \mu\text{g}}{\text{wt} \times \text{day}} = \frac{50 \mu\text{g}}{\text{day}} \times \frac{1}{1000} \times \frac{1500}{\text{wt}}$$

Step 5: Complete the required mathematical operations.

$$\frac{x\,\mu g}{wt \times day} = \frac{75\,\mu g}{day \times wt}$$

Since the total dose is 75 μg, the three doses are:

Dose 1 = 1/2(75 μg) = 37.50 μg
Dose 2 = 1/4(75 μg) = 18.75 μg
Dose 3 = 1/4(75 μg) = 18.75 μg
Total dose = 75.00 μg

▶ SOLVED PRACTICE PROBLEMS

1. The recommended dose of erythromycin is 5 mg/kg t.i.d. How many mg should a 40-kg child receive in a 24-hour period?

$$\frac{x\,mg}{wt \times day} = \frac{5\,mg}{kg \times dose} \times \frac{40\,kg}{wt} \times \frac{3\,doses}{1\,day}$$

▶ **Answer:** 600 mg

2. The recommended dose of aqueous penicillin G is 50,000 units/kg/d in 2 equally divided doses. For an infant weighing 4200 g, how many units per day would be recommended?

$$\frac{x\,U}{wt \times day} = \frac{50,000\,U}{kg \times day} \times \frac{1\,kg}{1000\,g} \times \frac{4200\,g}{wt}$$

▶ **Answer:** 210,000 U

3. The recommended dose of Macrodantin (nitrofurantoin) is 6 mg/kg q.i.d. How many mg would be given to a 40-lb child in one full day of therapy?

$$\frac{x\,mg}{wt \times day} = \frac{6\,mg}{kg \times dose} \times \frac{1\,kg}{2.2\,lb} \times \frac{40\,lb}{wt} \times \frac{4\,doses}{1\,day}$$

▶ **Answer:** 436 mg

4. The recommended dose of phenobarbital for a 2900 g neonate is 4 mg/kg given q12h. How much medication should the newborn receive in a 24-hour period?

$$\frac{x\,mg}{wt \times day} = \frac{4\,mg}{kg \times dose} \times \frac{1\,kg}{1000\,g} \times \frac{2900\,g}{wt} \times \frac{2\,doses}{1\,day}$$

▶ **Answer:** 23 mg

5. The recommended dose of Lasix (furosemide) is 2 mg/kg/d divided equally q8h. This child weighs 13 kg. What is the recommended total daily dose of Lasix?

$$\frac{x \text{ mg}}{\text{wt} \times \text{day}} = \frac{2 \text{ mg}}{\text{kg} \times \text{day}} \times \frac{13 \text{ kg}}{\text{wt}}$$

▸ **Answer:** 26 mg

▲ CALCULATING MAXIMUM AND MINIMUM PEDIATRIC DOSES

Many medication dosages for pediatric patients are recommended as a range rather than a single quantity per kilogram. For such medications both the minimum and maximum recommended dosages should be calculated to determine the effective dose range. The calculations are carried out in exactly the same way as those for determination of a single dose or total daily dose.

Example 7.7: The recommended dose of Aminophylline (theophylline) is 2–5 mg/kg/dose. Determine the minimum and maximum single doses for a 42-kg child.

Part 1: Minimum Dose

Step 1: State the problem in equation form.

$$\frac{x \text{ mg}}{\text{wt} \times \text{dose}} = \frac{2 \text{ mg}}{\text{kg} \times \text{dose}}$$

Step 2: Identify the conversion factor needed to convert from mg/kg/dose to mg/wt/dose. The information needed from the problem to identify the conversion factor is: wt = 42 kg.

Step 3: Put into the equation the form of the conversion factor that will cancel the unwanted labels and leave only the desired labels on both sides of the equal sign.

$$\frac{x \text{ mg}}{\text{wt} \times \text{dose}} = \frac{2 \text{ mg}}{\text{kg} \times \text{dose}} \times \frac{42 \text{ kg}}{\text{wt}}$$

Step 4: Cancel the labels that appear in both the numerator and the denominator on the same side of the equal sign.

$$\frac{x \text{ mg}}{\text{wt} \times \text{dose}} = \frac{2 \text{ mg}}{\text{dose}} \times \frac{42}{\text{wt}}$$

Step 5: Complete the required mathematical operations.

$$\frac{x \text{ mg}}{\text{wt} \times \text{dose}} = \frac{84 \text{ mg}}{\text{dose} \times \text{wt}}$$

Therefore, 84 mg is the minimum dose for a 42-kg child.

Part 2: Maximum Dose

To calculate the maximum dose, substitute 5 mg/kg/dose for 2 mg/kg/dose to give:

$$\frac{x \text{ mg}}{\text{wt} \times \text{dose}} = \frac{5 \text{ mg}}{\text{kg} \times \text{dose}} \times \frac{42 \text{ kg}}{\text{wt}}$$

$$\frac{x\,\text{mg}}{\text{wt} \times \text{dose}} = \frac{210\,\text{mg}}{\text{dose} \times \text{wt}}$$

Therefore, 210 mg is the maximum dose for a 42-kg child.

► SOLVED PRACTICE PROBLEMS

1. The recommended dose of Benadryl (diphenhydramine) is 4–6 mg/kg/day given in 4 equally divided doses. The medication is supplied in an elixir form with 12.5 mg per 5 ml. What are the minimum and maximum number of ml to give to a 12-kg infant?

Minimum: $\dfrac{x\,\text{ml}}{\text{wt} \times \text{dose}} = \dfrac{4\,\text{mg}}{\text{kg} \times \text{day}} \times \dfrac{12\,\text{kg}}{\text{wt}} \times \dfrac{1\,\text{day}}{4\,\text{doses}} \times \dfrac{5\,\text{ml}}{12.5\,\text{mg}}$

Maximum: $\dfrac{x\,\text{ml}}{\text{wt} \times \text{dose}} = \dfrac{6\,\text{mg}}{\text{kg} \times \text{day}} \times \dfrac{12\,\text{kg}}{\text{wt}} \times \dfrac{1\,\text{day}}{4\,\text{doses}} \times \dfrac{5\,\text{ml}}{12.5\,\text{mg}}$

► **Answer:** Min = 4.8 ml; Max = 7.2 ml

2. The recommended dose of Demerol (meperidine) is 0.6–1.5 mg/kg as an analgesic dose q6h. The medication is supplied 50 mg per cc. Determine the minimum and maximum cc dose for an 18-kg child.

Minimum: $\dfrac{x\,\text{cc}}{\text{wt} \times \text{dose}} = \dfrac{0.6\,\text{mg}}{\text{kg} \times \text{dose}} \times \dfrac{18\,\text{kg}}{\text{wt}} \times \dfrac{1\,\text{cc}}{50\,\text{mg}}$

Maximum: $\dfrac{x\,\text{cc}}{\text{wt} \times \text{dose}} = \dfrac{1.5\,\text{mg}}{\text{kg} \times \text{dose}} \times \dfrac{18\,\text{kg}}{\text{wt}} \times \dfrac{1\,\text{cc}}{50\,\text{mg}}$

► **Answer:** Min = 0.22 cc; Max = 0.54 cc

3. The recommended loading dose of Dilantin (phenytoin) is 15–20 mg/kg for the single dose. Calculate the minimum and maximum loading dose for an infant weighing 22 lb.

Minimum: $\dfrac{x\,\text{mg}}{\text{wt} \times \text{dose}} = \dfrac{15\,\text{mg}}{\text{kg} \times \text{dose}} \times \dfrac{1\,\text{kg}}{2.2\,\text{lb}} \times \dfrac{22\,\text{lb}}{\text{wt}}$

Maximum: $\dfrac{x\,\text{mg}}{\text{wt} \times \text{dose}} = \dfrac{20\,\text{mg}}{\text{kg} \times \text{dose}} \times \dfrac{1\,\text{kg}}{2.2\,\text{lb}} \times \dfrac{22\,\text{lb}}{\text{wt}}$

► **Answer:** Min = 150 mg; Max = 200 mg

4. The recommended dose of chloral hydrate is 20–30 mg/kg. The child weighs 36 lb, and the concentration of the medication is 500 mg per 5 cc. Determine the minimum and maximum number of cc per dose.

Minimum: $\dfrac{x\,\text{cc}}{\text{wt} \times \text{dose}} = \dfrac{20\,\text{mg}}{\text{kg} \times \text{dose}} \times \dfrac{1\,\text{kg}}{2.2\,\text{lb}} \times \dfrac{36\,\text{lb}}{\text{wt}} \times \dfrac{5\,\text{cc}}{500\,\text{mg}}$

Maximum: $\dfrac{x\,\text{cc}}{\text{wt} \times \text{dose}} = \dfrac{30\,\text{mg}}{\text{kg} \times \text{dose}} \times \dfrac{1\,\text{kg}}{2.2\,\text{lb}} \times \dfrac{36\,\text{lb}}{\text{wt}} \times \dfrac{5\,\text{cc}}{500\,\text{mg}}$

► **Answer:** Min = 3.3 cc; Max = 4.9 cc

5. The recommended dose of Compazine (prochlorperazine) is 0.25–0.35 mg/kg/d divided equally q8h. The weight of the child is 50 lb. Determine the minimum and maximum doses.

Minimum: $\dfrac{x \text{ mg}}{\text{wt} \times \text{dose}} = \dfrac{0.25 \text{ mg}}{\text{kg} \times \text{day}} \times \dfrac{1 \text{ kg}}{2.2 \text{ lb}} \times \dfrac{50 \text{ lb}}{\text{wt}} \times \dfrac{1 \text{ day}}{3 \text{ doses}}$

Maximum: $\dfrac{x \text{ mg}}{\text{wt} \times \text{dose}} = \dfrac{0.35 \text{ mg}}{\text{kg} \times \text{day}} \times \dfrac{1 \text{ kg}}{2.2 \text{ lb}} \times \dfrac{50 \text{ lb}}{\text{wt}} \times \dfrac{1 \text{ day}}{3 \text{ doses}}$

▸ **Answer:** Min = 1.9 mg; Max = 2.7 mg

◢ DETERMINATION OF A REASONABLE PEDIATRIC DOSE

Prior to administration of a pediatric drug, it is necessary to determine if an ordered dose of medication is reasonable based on the body weight of the patient and the manufacturer's recommended dose. It is important to calculate both the recommended single dose and the recommended total daily dose. If an ordered dose exceeds a recommended dose, further clarification of the dose should be sought from the physician.

The steps to follow in this process are:

1. Calculate the recommended single dose.
2. Calculate the recommended total daily dose.
3. Calculate the total daily dose ordered.
4. Compare the recommended and the ordered doses.

Example 7.8: The order is chloramphenicol 600 mg q8h. The child weighs 18.3 kg. The recommended dose is 100 mg/kg/d divided equally q6h. Determine if the ordered dose is reasonable.

Calculate the Recommended Single Dose:

$$\frac{x \text{ mg}}{\text{wt} \times \text{dose}} = \frac{100 \text{ mg}}{\text{kg} \times \text{day}} \times \frac{18.3 \text{ kg}}{\text{wt}} \times \frac{1 \text{ day}}{4 \text{ doses}}$$

$$\frac{x \text{ mg}}{\text{wt} \times \text{dose}} = \frac{457.5 \text{ mg}}{\text{kg} \times \text{dose}}$$

The recommended single dose for an 18.3 kg child is 458 mg.

Calculate the Recommended Total Daily Dose:

$$\frac{x \text{ mg}}{\text{wt} \times \text{day}} = \frac{100 \text{ mg}}{\text{kg} \times \text{day}} \times \frac{18.3 \text{ kg}}{\text{wt}}$$

$$\frac{x \text{ mg}}{\text{wt} \times \text{day}} = \frac{1830 \text{ mg}}{\text{day} \times \text{wt}}$$

The recommended total daily dose for an 18.3 kg child is 1830 mg.

Calculate the Total Daily Dose Ordered:
Recall that the physician's order is 600 mg q8h, or three times in 24 hours.

$$\frac{x\,\text{mg}}{\text{day}} = \frac{600\,\text{mg}}{\text{dose}} \times \frac{3\,\text{doses}}{1\,\text{day}}$$

$$\frac{x\,\text{mg}}{\text{day}} = \frac{1800\,\text{mg}}{\text{day}}$$

The total daily dose ordered is 1800 mg.

Compare the Recommended and the Ordered Doses:

DOSES	RECOMMENDED	ORDERED
Single	458 mg	600 mg
Total daily	1830 mg	1800 mg
Doses/day	4	3

The ordered dose of 600 mg q8h *does exceed* the recommended single dose even though it does not exceed the recommended total daily dose. Verification of the order is necessary prior to administration of the medication.

Example 7.9: A 55-lb child is to receive Dilantin (phenytoin) 75 mg q12h. The recommended dose range is 4–8 mg/kg/24 h in single or divided doses. (The reasonable dose should fall within the recommended dose range.) Determine if the ordered dose is reasonable.

Calculate the Recommended Single Dose:
It is necessary to determine the recommended range. Therefore, both minimum and maximum doses are calculated.

Part 1: Minimum Dose

$$\frac{x\,\text{mg}}{\text{wt} \times \text{dose}} = \frac{4\,\text{mg}}{\text{kg} \times \text{day}} \times \frac{1\,\text{kg}}{2.2\,\text{lb}} \times \frac{55\,\text{lb}}{\text{wt}} \times \frac{1\,\text{day}}{2\,\text{doses}}$$

$$\frac{x\,\text{mg}}{\text{wt} \times \text{dose}} = \frac{50\,\text{mg}}{\text{wt} \times \text{dose}}$$

The minimum single dose is 50 mg.

Part 2: Maximum Dose

$$\frac{x\,\text{mg}}{\text{wt} \times \text{dose}} = \frac{8\,\text{mg}}{\text{kg} \times \text{day}} \times \frac{1\,\text{kg}}{2.2\,\text{lb}} \times \frac{55\,\text{lb}}{\text{wt}} \times \frac{1\,\text{day}}{2\,\text{doses}}$$

$$\frac{x\,\text{mg}}{\text{wt} \times \text{dose}} = \frac{100\,\text{mg}}{\text{wt} \times \text{dose}}$$

The maximum single dose is 100 mg.

Calculate the Recommended Total Daily Dose:

Part 1: Minimum Dose

$$\frac{x\,\text{mg}}{\text{wt} \times \text{day}} = \frac{4\,\text{mg}}{\text{kg} \times \text{day}} \times \frac{1\,\text{kg}}{2.2\,\text{lb}} \times \frac{55\,\text{lb}}{\text{wt}}$$

$$\frac{x\,\text{mg}}{\text{wt} \times \text{day}} = \frac{100\,\text{mg}}{\text{day} \times \text{wt}}$$

The minimum total daily dose is 100 mg.

Part 2: Maximum Dose

$$\frac{x \text{ mg}}{\text{wt} \times \text{day}} = \frac{8 \text{ mg}}{\text{kg} \times \text{day}} \times \frac{1 \text{ kg}}{2.2 \text{ lb}} \times \frac{55 \text{ lb}}{\text{wt}}$$

$$\frac{x \text{ mg}}{\text{wt} \times \text{day}} = \frac{200 \text{ mg}}{\text{day} \times \text{wt}}$$

The maximum total daily dose is 200 mg.

Calculate the Total Daily Dose Ordered:
Recall that the physician's order is 75 mg q12h, or 2 times a day.

$$\frac{x \text{ mg}}{\text{day}} = \frac{75 \text{ mg}}{\text{dose}} \times \frac{2 \text{ doses}}{1 \text{ day}}$$

$$\frac{x \text{ mg}}{\text{day}} = \frac{150 \text{ mg}}{\text{day}}$$

The total daily dose ordered is 150 mg.

Compare the Recommended and the Ordered Doses:

DOSES	RECOMMENDED	ORDERED
Single	50–100 mg	75 mg
Total daily	100–200 mg	150 mg
Doses/day	2	2

The ordered dose of 75 mg q12h falls within the recommended dose range for a 55-lb child.

▶ SOLVED PRACTICE PROBLEMS

1. The physician has ordered codeine IM 10 mg q6h prn for a child who weighs 35 lb. The recommended dose is 3 mg/kg/day in 4 equally divided doses. Determine if the ordered dose is reasonable.

    A. The recommended single dose is 12 mg.

    $$\frac{x \text{ mg}}{\text{wt} \times \text{dose}} = \frac{3 \text{ mg}}{\text{kg} \times \text{day}} \times \frac{1 \text{ kg}}{2.2 \text{ lb}} \times \frac{35 \text{ lb}}{\text{wt}} \times \frac{1 \text{ day}}{4 \text{ doses}}$$

    B. The recommended total daily dose is 48 mg.

    $$\frac{x \text{ mg}}{\text{wt} \times \text{day}} = \frac{3 \text{ mg}}{\text{kg} \times \text{day}} \times \frac{1 \text{ kg}}{2.2 \text{ lb}} \times \frac{35 \text{ lb}}{\text{wt}}$$

C. The total daily dose ordered is 40 mg.

$$\frac{x \text{ mg}}{\text{day}} = \frac{10 \text{ mg}}{\text{dose}} \times \frac{4 \text{ doses}}{1 \text{ day}}$$

▶ **Answer:** The ordered dose does not exceed the manufacturer's recommended dose.

2. The physician's order is Unipen (nafcillin) 350 mg PO q4h for a 28.5 kg child. The recommended dose is 50 mg/kg/d in 4 equally divided doses. Determine if the ordered dose is reasonable.

A. The recommended single dose is 356 mg.

$$\frac{x \text{ mg}}{\text{wt} \times \text{dose}} = \frac{50 \text{ mg}}{\text{kg} \times \text{day}} \times \frac{28.5 \text{ kg}}{\text{wt}} \times \frac{1 \text{ day}}{4 \text{ doses}}$$

B. The recommended total daily dose is 1425 mg.

$$\frac{x \text{ mg}}{\text{wt} \times \text{day}} = \frac{50 \text{ mg}}{\text{kg} \times \text{day}} \times \frac{28.5 \text{ kg}}{\text{wt}}$$

C. The total daily dose ordered is 2100 mg.

$$\frac{x \text{ mg}}{\text{day}} = \frac{350 \text{ mg}}{\text{dose}} \times \frac{6 \text{ doses}}{1 \text{ day}}$$

▶ **Answer:** The ordered dose *does exceed* the manufacturer's recommended total daily dose. Verification of this order should be sought prior to administration of the medication.

3. The order is to give propylthiouracil 125 mg PO t.i.d. to a 96-lb child. The recommended dose is 7 mg/kg/d in 3 equally divided doses. Determine if the ordered dose is reasonable.

A. The recommended single dose is 102 mg.

$$\frac{x \text{ mg}}{\text{wt} \times \text{dose}} = \frac{7 \text{ mg}}{\text{kg} \times \text{day}} \times \frac{1 \text{ kg}}{2.2 \text{ lb}} \times \frac{96 \text{ lb}}{\text{wt}} \times \frac{1 \text{ day}}{3 \text{ doses}}$$

B. The recommended total daily dose is 305 mg.

$$\frac{x \text{ mg}}{\text{wt} \times \text{day}} = \frac{7 \text{ mg}}{\text{kg} \times \text{day}} \times \frac{1 \text{ kg}}{2.2 \text{ lb}} \times \frac{96 \text{ lb}}{\text{wt}}$$

C. The total daily dose ordered is 375 mg.

$$\frac{x \text{ mg}}{\text{day}} = \frac{125 \text{ mg}}{\text{dose}} \times \frac{3 \text{ doses}}{\text{day}}$$

▶ **Answer:** The ordered dose *does exceed* both the manufacturer's recommended single and total daily doses. Verification of this order should be sought prior to administration of the medication.

4. The physician's order is to give a 2800 g neonate chloramphenicol 35 mg IV, q6h. The maximum recommended dose is 50 mg/kg/d in 4 equally divided doses. Determine if the ordered dose is reasonable.

A. The recommended single dose is 35 mg.

$$\frac{x\,\text{mg}}{\text{wt} \times \text{dose}} = \frac{50\,\text{mg}}{\text{kg} \times \text{day}} \times \frac{1\,\text{kg}}{1000\,\text{g}} \times \frac{2800\,\text{g}}{\text{wt}} \times \frac{1\,\text{day}}{4\,\text{doses}}$$

B. The recommended total daily dose is 140 mg.

$$\frac{x\,\text{mg}}{\text{wt} \times \text{day}} = \frac{50\,\text{mg}}{\text{kg} \times \text{day}} \times \frac{1\,\text{kg}}{1000\,\text{g}} \times \frac{2800\,\text{g}}{\text{wt}}$$

C. The total daily dose ordered is 140 mg.

$$\frac{x\,\text{mg}}{\text{day}} = \frac{35\,\text{mg}}{\text{dose}} \times \frac{4\,\text{doses}}{1\,\text{day}}$$

▶ **Answer:** The ordered dose does not exceed the manufacturer's recommended dose.

5. The maintenance dose of digoxin ordered for a 3200-g neonate is 50 μg b.i.d. The recommended dose is 12.5–16.7 μg/kg/d divided equally b.i.d. Determine if the ordered dose is reasonable.

A. The maximum recommended single dose is 26.72 μg.

$$\frac{x\,\mu\text{g}}{\text{wt} \times \text{dose}} = \frac{16.7\,\mu\text{g}}{\text{kg} \times \text{day}} \times \frac{1\,\text{kg}}{1000\,\text{g}} \times \frac{3200\,\text{g}}{\text{wt}} \times \frac{1\,\text{day}}{2\,\text{doses}}$$

B. The maximum recommended total daily dose is 53.44 μg.

$$\frac{x\,\mu\text{g}}{\text{wt} \times \text{day}} = \frac{16.7\,\mu\text{g}}{\text{kg} \times \text{day}} \times \frac{1\,\text{kg}}{1000\,\text{g}} \times \frac{3200\,\text{g}}{\text{wt}}$$

C. The total daily dose ordered is 100 μg.

$$\frac{x\,\mu\text{g}}{\text{day}} = \frac{50\,\mu\text{g}}{\text{dose}} \times \frac{2\,\text{doses}}{1\,\text{day}}$$

▶ **Answer:** The ordered dose *does exceed* both the manufacturer's recommended single and total daily dose. Verification of this order should be sought prior to administration of the medication.

CASE STUDIES

► Case Six

E.F. is a 20-month-old child admitted with a 2-day history of anorexia, elevated temperature, and irritability. E.F. weighs 26.4 lb. His current medical diagnosis is meningitis. Among his medical orders are: diet as tolerated; Tylenol elixir 2 cc for temp ≥101F; neuro checks q2h; seizure precautions; IV of 5% dextrose and RL at 30 cc/hr; and Polycillin-N 350 mg IVPB q4h.

Polycillin-N is sent from the pharmacy in a vial with the following label:

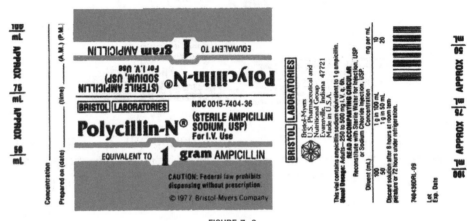

FIGURE 7–3.
(Used with permission of Bristol Meyer Squibb Company.)

The manufacturer's medication insert states that the recommended parenteral dose of Polycillin-N for bacterial meningitis is: "Adults and children: 150 to 200 mg/kg/d in equally divided doses every 3–4 hours."

Refer to the medication label and insert as needed to answer the following questions.

1. How many kilograms does the patient weigh?
2. What is the minimum recommended q4h dose for this child?
3. What is the maximum recommended q4h dose for this child?
4. What is the minimum recommended daily dose?
5. What is the maximum recommended daily dose?
6. Does the ordered single dose fall within the recommended range?
7. How much Polycillin-N is the patient receiving per day?
8. Does the ordered daily dose fall within the recommended range?

For answers to Case Study Six, see page 135.

► Case Seven

C.C., a 40-lb child, is admitted with a secondary bacterial infection of the lung related to influenza. The current medical orders include: bed rest, O_2 at 40% per tent, IPPB treatment q6h, and Tegopen (cloxacillin) 200 mg PO q6h.

Tegopen is sent from the pharmacy with the following label:

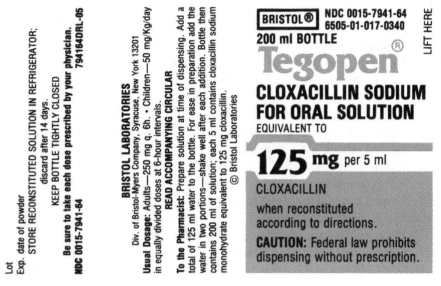

FIGURE 7–4.

Refer to the medication label to answer the following questions:

1. How many mg does each 5 ml of Tegopen contain?
2. What is the manufacturer's recommended dose in mg/kg/d?
3. What is the recommended dose for this child per day?
4. What is the recommended number of mg per dose?
5. Does the ordered dose exceed the recommended dose for an adult?

For answers to Case Study Seven, see page 135.

▶ SELF-TEST

1. The recommended dose of Lasix (furosemide) is 2 mg/kg/d divided q8h. What is the recommended single q8h dose for a 38.8 lb child?
2. The physician ordered the neonatal digitalizing dose of digoxin, 50 μg/kg, for an infant weighing 3.75 lb. The medication is to be given in three doses divided 1/2, 1/4, 1/4. Determine each of the three doses.
3. The recommended dose of Mysoline (primidone) is 10–25 mg/kg/d divided b.i.d. Determine the maximum recommended single dose for a 40 lb child.
4. The recommended maintenance dose of Dilantin (phenytoin) is 4–8 mg/kg/d divided equally q12h. The medication is supplied 125 mg per 5 cc. The child weighs 15 kg. Determine the maximum number of cc recommended per dose.

Continued next page

▶ Self-Test Continued

5. The recommended dose of penicillin G is 250,000 units/kg/d divided in equal doses q4h. The medication is available as 1,000,000 units per 10 ml. The infant weighs 12.5 lb. Determine the number of cc recommended per dose.

6. The recommended dose of Tylenol (acetaminophen) is 25 mg/kg/d q6h. Determine the total daily dose for a 10 kg infant.

7. The recommended dose of tetracycline is 50 mg/kg/24 h divided into 4 equal doses. Determine the total daily dose for a 110 lb child.

8. The recommended dose of Garamycin (gentamicin) is 7.5 mg/kg/d divided equally q8h. Determine the total daily dose for a 9-lb, 8-oz infant.

9. The recommended dose of Vistaril (hydroxyzine) is 4 mg/kg/24 h in 3 equal doses. Determine the total daily dose for a 48 lb child.

10. The recommended dose of Keflex (cephalexin) is 25–50 mg/kg every 12 hours. Determine the maximum total daily dose for a 30 lb child.

11. The recommended dose range for erythromycin is 20–50 mg/kg/d divided equally q6h. Determine the minimum and maximum doses for a 5 kg infant.

12. The recommended single dose of aminophylline is 2–5 mg/kg/dose. Calculate the minimum and maximum dose for a 55 lb child.

13. Using the data from problem 12, calculate the minimum and maximum number of cc per dose if the medication is supplied in ampules with 250 mg per 10 cc.

14. The recommended oral dose of Ceclor (cefaclor) is 40–60 mg/kg/d divided q6h in equal doses. For a 45.5 lb child, determine the minimum and maximum doses.

15. The physician ordered sodium bicarbonate, 5 mEq/kg/dose, for a 1900-g neonate. The recommended neonatal dose is 1–3 mEq/kg/dose. Determine if the ordered dose is reasonable.

16. The physician ordered Lasix (furosemide) stat, 3 mg IV push, for a 4500-g neonate. The recommended neonatal dose is 1 mg/kg/dose. Determine if the ordered dose is reasonable.

17. The physician ordered penicillin G 125,000 units IV q6h for a 13.2 lb infant. The recommended dose is 20,000–50,000 units/kg/day in 4 equal doses. Determine if the ordered dose is reasonable.

18. The physician ordered Demerol (meperidine) 25 mg q6h prn for a 38 lb child. The recommended dose is 1 mg/kg/dose q4–6h. Determine if the ordered dose is reasonable.

19. The physician ordered Vibramycin (doxycycline) 100 mg q12h for a 31 kg child. The recommended dose is 5 mg/kg/d divided in 2 equal doses. Determine if the ordered dose is reasonable.

20. The physician ordered phenobarbital gr i q6h for a 30-kg child. The recommended dose is 2 mg/kg/dose q6h. Determine if the ordered dose is reasonable.

For answers to the self-test, see page 135.

1. 12 kg
2. 300 mg
3. 400 mg
4. 1800 mg
5. 2400 mg
6. Yes
7. 2100 mg
8. Yes

1. 125 mg
2. 50 mg/kg/d
3. 909.1 mg
4. 227.3 mg
5. No, it does not exceed the recommended dose for an adult.

1. 12 mg
2. Dose 1 (1/2 dose) = 42.6 μg; dose 2 (1/4 dose) = 21.3 μg; dose 3 (1/4 dose) = 21.3 μg
3. 227 mg
4. 2.4 cc
5. 2.4 cc
6. 250 mg
7. 2500 mg
8. 32 mg
9. 87 mg
10. 1364 mg
11. Min = 25 mg, max = 63 mg
12. Min = 50 mg, max = 125 mg
13. Min = 2 cc, max = 5 cc
14. Min = 207 mg, max = 310 mg
15. Ordered dose does not exceed recommended dose.
16. Ordered dose does not exceed recommended dose.
17. Ordered dose *does exceed* the recommended dose.
18. Ordered dose *does exceed* the recommended dose.
19. Ordered dose *does exceed* the recommended dose.
20. Ordered dose does not exceed the recommended dose.

Intravenous Fluids

8

8

▲ OBJECTIVES

Upon completion of Chapter 8, the student will be able to:

► Consistently express the rate of an IV infusion, calculated in either drops per minute or milliliters per hour, in whole numbers only.

► Correctly calculate the rate of infusion in drops per minute or in milliliters per hour of an IV solution for general fluid replacement given any drop factor and the amount of fluid to be infused over a given time.

► Correctly calculate the rate of infusion in drops per minute or in milliliters per hour of blood, blood products, and plasma expanders given any drop factor and the amount to be infused over a given time.

► Correctly calculate the amount of KCl to be added to an IV solution to administer the dose prescribed in the proper concentration.

▲ INTRODUCTION TO ADMINISTRATION OF INTRAVENOUS FLUIDS

The physician orders the administration of intravenous fluids by specifying both the type and volume of fluid to be given and the rate of administration of the fluid. The rate is normally specified in terms of a certain number of milliliters over a certain number of hours.

Intravenous solutions are administered through various types of infusion sets. Each set is made of tubing that delivers a specific number of drops of IV fluid per milliliter. It is the nurse's responsibility to calculate how many drops per minute are required to deliver the ordered amount of IV fluid in the time indicated.

Intravenous fluids and medications are injected directly into the bloodstream. As a result, medications given by this route act rapidly. Common sites for the administration of IV fluids include the veins of the hands, forearms, feet, neck, and scalp; the subclavian vein may also be used. Many different types of intravenous fluids are available for administration. Solutions containing dextrose and/or saline are most commonly ordered by physicians.

Sterile equipment must be used when administering intravenous fluids and medications. Basic equipment includes the following:

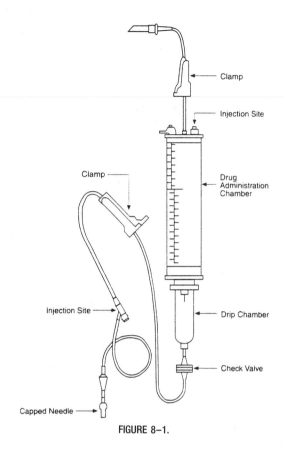

FIGURE 8–1.

1. Intravenous needle or catheter
2. Administration set or tubing
   A. Macrodrop tubing delivers 10, 15, or 20 drops per ml (gtts/ml)
   B. Minidrop (microdrop) tubing delivers 60 drops per ml (gtts/ml)
3. Container of IV fluid

An accessory item sometimes used in the administration of IV fluids is a volume control set such as a Buretrol shown in Figure 8–1. Volume control sets are usually minidrop sets (delivering 60 gtts/ml), which facilitate the administration of small amounts of fluid. Additionally, mechanical IV flow regulators may also be used.

Health care facilities typically stock one brand of macrodrop IV tubing and one brand of minidrop IV tubing. The decision to use either macrodrop or minidrop tubing is often left to the nurse. In the absence of policies to guide decisions, nurses typically use minidrop tubing when the amount of fluid to infuse needs to be infused slowly.

exercise

▲ INTRAVENOUS FLUID TUBING

Importance of Knowing the Correct Drop Factor: The drop factor for
an IV infusion set will always be printed on the packaging, as can be seen in Figure 8–2. Nurses must be certain of the drop factor of the particular tubing being used to avoid infusing too much or too little fluid over a given time.

Using the choices given, which mistake would be made in each of the following cases:

Choices:
A. 1/2 as much fluid given as ordered
B. 1 1/2 times as much fluid given as ordered
C. 2 times as much fluid given as ordered

1. A nurse mistakenly assumed an IV tubing had a drop factor of 20 gtts/ml when it actually was 10 gtts/ml.
2. A nurse mistakenly assumed an IV tubing had a drop factor of 15 gtts/ml when it actually was 10 gtts/ml.

2C5401 s

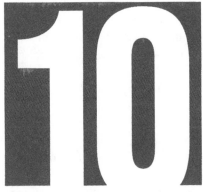

Baxter

**Basic
Solution Set**

Flashball® Device

10

10 drops approx. 1 mL

1.8 m (70") long

*Sterile, nonpyrogenic fluid path

Caution: Federal (USA) law restricts this device to sale by or on order of a physician.

FIGURE 8–2.

3. A nurse mistakenly assumed an IV tubing had a drop factor of 10 gtts/ml when it actually was 20 gtts/ml.

Answers: C; B; A

> ► **alert:**
>
> Use minidrop tubing to minimize the risk of infusing IV fluid too rapidly.

> ► **critical decision point:**
>
> A nurse finds the following orders written for three different patients. Read each order and determine if minidrop tubing would be the most appropriate to use.
> Patient 1: *IV of 1000 cc 5% dextrose in 0.45% sodium chloride every 8 h*
> Patient 2: *IV of 100 cc of 5% dextrose with 60 mEq KCl over 6 h*
> Patient 3: *IV to keep vein open with 5% dextrose*

> ► **decision/action:**
>
> Patient 1: An infusion of 3000 cc in 24 hours would not be considered a slow infusion; therefore, the nurse could elect to *use either* a macrodrop or minidrop tubing. Patient 2: To infuse 100 cc over 6 hours requires a carefully regulated, slow infusion; therefore, the nurse should *use only* minidrop tubing. Patient 3: Any order to keep a vein open indicates a slow infusion; therefore, the nurse would *normally use* minidrop tubing.

▲ INTRODUCTION TO IV CALCULATIONS

Intravenous infusion rates can be calculated in terms of the number of drops per minute (gtts/min) or the number of milliliters per hour (ml/h) needed to administer the fluid as ordered by the physician. When rates are calculated in drops per minute, it is necessary to know how many drops per ml are delivered by the IV tubing being used. This characteristic of the IV tubing, referred to as the drop factor, varies with each manufacturer.

In this chapter, the drop factor of the tubing being used is specified in any problem in which the rate is to be calculated in terms of drops per minute. All rates are calculated by the dimensional analysis method of problem solving discussed in Chapter 2. The application of the method to the calculation of IV rates is illustrated below.

Rounding answers. When calculating intravenous infusion rates in either drops per minute or milliliters per hour, answers are always rounded to whole numbers. Decimal numbers are not clinically feasible when working with IV rates.

Example 8.1: The order is to infuse 1000 cc of Ringer's lactate solution over the next 8 hours. Determine the rate in drops per minute using an infusion set with a drop factor of 15 drops per cc.

► **Rules of Problem Solving by Dimensional Analysis**

RULE 1 ► One side of an equation can be multiplied by an appropriate conversion factor without changing the value of the equation.

▶ Application of Rule 1

When calculating intravenous fluid rates, the drop factor is considered to be a conversion factor. In the example given above, the administration set has a drop factor of 15 drops per 1 cc. Therefore, the conversion factor is:1 cc = 15 gtts. The conversion factor can be put into the problem in either of two possible forms:

$$\frac{15 \text{ gtts}}{1 \text{ cc}} \quad \text{or} \quad \frac{1 \text{ cc}}{15 \text{ gtts}}$$

The problem is correctly set up when all labels cancel from both the numerator and the denominator except the labels desired in the answer.

◀ RULE 2

▶ Application of Rule 2

1. In the problem given, the question asked is how many drops per minute will equal 1000 cubic centimeters in 8 hours.
2. Stated in an equation form, the problem is:

$$\frac{x \text{ gtts}}{\text{min}} = \frac{1000 \text{ cc}}{8 \text{ h}}$$

3. Since the unit of time in the answer is minute, but the unit of time in the physician's order is hour, a conversion factor relating minute and hour is needed. That conversion factor is 1 hour equals 60 minutes.

   The two conversion factors, 1 hour = 60 minutes and15 gtts = 1 cc, are put into the equation as fractions. The form of each fraction used is that which will cancel the unwanted labels (cubic centimeters and hours) and leave only the desired labels (drops and minutes) on both sides of the equal sign.

$$\frac{x \text{ gtts}}{\text{min}} = \frac{1000 \text{ cc}}{8 \text{ h}} \times \frac{15 \text{ gtts}}{1 \text{ cc}} \times \frac{1 \text{ h}}{60 \text{ min}}$$

   The equation can now be read: x drops per minute equal 1000 cubic centimeters per 8 hours when it is true that there are 15 drops per 1 cubic centimeter, and when it is true that in 1 hour there are 60 minutes.

4. Cancel labels that appear in both the numerator and denominator on the same side of the equal sign.

$$\frac{x \text{ gtts}}{\text{min}} = \frac{1000}{8} \times \frac{15 \text{ gtts}}{1} \times \frac{1}{60 \text{ min}}$$

5. Completing the required mathematical operations gives:

$$\frac{x \text{ gtts}}{\text{min}} = \frac{1000 \times 15 \text{ gtts} \times 1}{8 \times 1 \times 60 \text{ min}} = \frac{31.3 \text{ gtts}}{\text{min}}$$

   The answer must be rounded to a whole number. Therefore, the rate of the IV is 31 gtts/min.

The method of problem solving by dimensional analysis illustrated above is used throughout this chapter. For simplicity the method is reduced to the same five-step procedure used in previous chapters.

▲ GENERAL FLUID REPLACEMENT

Example 8.2: The physician has ordered 1000 cc of 5% dextrose to be given over the next 12 hours. The drop factor of the tubing is 60 gtts/cc. Determine the rate of the IV in gtts/min and cc/h.

Part 1: Find Drops per Minute

Step 1:   State the problem in equation form.

$$\frac{x \text{ gtts}}{\text{min}} = \frac{1000 \text{ cc}}{12 \text{ h}}$$

Step 2:   Identify the conversion factors needed to convert from cubic centimeters per hour to drops per minute.

Two conversion factors are used:

A. Convert from cubic centimeters to drops.

1 cc = 60 gtts

B. Convert from hours to minutes.

1 h = 60 min

Step 3:   Put into the equation the form of the conversion factor that will cancel the unwanted labels and leave only the desired labels on both sides of the equal sign.

$$\frac{x \text{ gtts}}{\text{min}} = \frac{1000 \text{ cc}}{12 \text{ h}} \times \frac{60 \text{ gtts}}{1 \text{ cc}} \times \frac{1 \text{ h}}{60 \text{ min}}$$

Step 4:   Cancel the labels that appear in both the numerator and the denominator on the same side of the equal sign.

$$\frac{x \text{ gtts}}{\text{min}} = \frac{1000}{12} \times \frac{60 \text{ gtts}}{1} \times \frac{1}{60 \text{ min}}$$

Step 5:   Complete the required mathematical operations.

$$\frac{x \text{ gtts}}{\text{min}} = \frac{83.3 \text{ gtts}}{\text{min}}$$

The answer *must* be rounded to a whole number. Therefore, the rate of the IV is 83 gtts/min.

Part 2: Find Cubic Centimeters per Hour

Step 1:   State the problem in equation form.

$$\frac{x \text{ cc}}{\text{h}} = \frac{1000 \text{ cc}}{12 \text{ h}}$$

Step 2:   No conversion factors are needed since the labels required in the answer, cubic centimeters and hours, are the only labels in the problem.

$$\frac{x \text{ cc}}{\text{h}} = \frac{1000 \text{ cc}}{12 \text{ h}} = \frac{83.3 \text{ cc}}{\text{h}}$$

The answer *must* be rounded to a whole number. Therefore, the rate of IV is 83 cc/h.

When using infusion sets with a drop factor of 60 drops per cubic centimeter (minidrop sets), it is always true that the numerical value of cubic centimeters per hour will equal the numerical value of drops per minute. In Example 8.2 a minidrop set is used and the rate calculated is 83 gtts/min and 83 cc/h. As illustrated below, this is a result of using two conversion factors that each contain the number 60 (60 gtts = 1 cc and 1 hr = 60 min) in the calculations.

Compare Part 1, Step 3, and Part 2, Step 1 of Example 8.2.

Part 1, Step 3:

$$\frac{x \text{ gtts}}{\text{min}} = \frac{1000 \text{ cc}}{12 \text{ h}} \times \frac{60 \text{ gtts}}{1 \text{ cc}} \times \frac{1 \text{ h}}{60 \text{ min}}$$

Cancel like labels and numbers to obtain

$$\frac{x \text{ gtts}}{\text{min}} = \frac{1000}{12} \times \frac{1 \text{ gtts}}{1} \times \frac{1}{\text{min}}$$

(*Note:* The two 60s cancel, leaving only the division of 1000 by 12 to equal 83.3 Part 2, Step 1.)

$$\frac{x \text{ cc}}{\text{h}} = \frac{1000 \text{ cc}}{12 \text{ h}}$$

(*Note:* This problem involves only the division of 1000 by 12 to equal 83.3.)

Example 8.3: The order is to administer 500 cc of 50% dextrose over the next 4 hours. The drop factor of the tubing is 10 gtts/cc. Determine the gtts/min and the cc/h.

Part 1: Find Drops per Minute

Step 1:   State the problem in equation form.

$$\frac{x \text{ gtts}}{\text{min}} = \frac{500 \text{ cc}}{4 \text{ h}}$$

Step 2:   Identify the conversion factors needed to convert from cubic centimeters per hour to drops per minute.

Two conversion factors are used:

A. Convert from cubic centimeters to drops.

   1 cc = 10 gtts

B. Convert from hours to minutes.

   1 h = 60 min

Step 3:   Put into the equation the form of each conversion factor that will cancel the unwanted labels and leave only the desired labels on both sides of the equal sign.

$$\frac{x \text{ gtts}}{\text{min}} = \frac{500 \text{ cc}}{4 \text{ h}} \times \frac{10 \text{ gtts}}{1 \text{ cc}} \times \frac{1 \text{ h}}{60 \text{ min}}$$

Step 4:   Cancel the labels that appear in both the numerator and the denominator on the same side of the equal sign.

$$\frac{x \text{ gtts}}{\text{min}} = \frac{500}{4} \times \frac{10 \text{ gtts}}{1} \times \frac{1}{60 \text{ min}}$$

Step 5: Complete the required mathematical operations.

$$\frac{x \text{ gtts}}{\text{min}} = \frac{20.8 \text{ gtts}}{\text{min}}$$

The answer *must* be rounded to a whole number. Therefore, the rate of IV is 21 gtts/min.

Part 2: Find Cubic Centimeters per Hour

Step 1: State the problem in equation form.

$$\frac{x \text{ cc}}{\text{h}} = \frac{500 \text{ cc}}{4 \text{ h}}$$

Step 2: No conversion factors are needed.

$$\frac{x \text{ cc}}{\text{h}} = \frac{500 \text{ cc}}{4 \text{ h}} = \frac{125 \text{ cc}}{\text{h}}$$

Therefore, the rate is 125 cc/h.

Example 8.4: The order is to give 3000 cc of 0.9% sodium chloride over the next 24 hours. The drop factor of the tubing is 15 gtts/cc. Determine the rate in gtts/min.

Step 1: State the problem in equation form.

$$\frac{x \text{ gtts}}{\text{min}} = \frac{3000 \text{ cc}}{24 \text{ h}}$$

Step 2: Identify the conversion factors needed to convert from cubic centimeters per hour to drops per minute.

Two conversion factors are used:

A. Convert from cubic centimeters to drops.

1 cc = 15 gtts

B. Convert from hours to minutes.

1 h = 60 min

Step 3: Put into the equation the form of each conversion factor that will cancel the unwanted labels and leave only the desired labels on both sides of the equal sign.

$$\frac{x \text{ gtts}}{\text{min}} = \frac{3000 \text{ cc}}{24 \text{ h}} \times \frac{15 \text{ gtts}}{1 \text{ cc}} \times \frac{1 \text{ h}}{60 \text{ min}}$$

Step 4: Cancel the labels that appear in both the numerator and the denominator on the same side of the equal sign.

$$\frac{x \text{ gtts}}{\text{min}} = \frac{3000}{24} \times \frac{15 \text{ gtts}}{1} \times \frac{1}{60 \text{ min}}$$

Step 5: Complete the required mathematical operations.

$$\frac{x \text{ gtts}}{\text{min}} = \frac{31.25 \text{ gtts}}{\text{min}}$$

Therefore, the rate is 31 gtts/min.

▶ SOLVED PRACTICE PROBLEMS

1. The patient is to receive 1000 cc of 0.45% sodium chloride over the next 10 hours. The drop factor of the tubing is 15 gtts/cc. Determine the rate in gtts/min.

$$\frac{x \text{ gtts}}{\text{min}} = \frac{1000 \text{ cc}}{10 \text{ h}} \times \frac{15 \text{ gtts}}{1 \text{ cc}} \times \frac{1 \text{ h}}{60 \text{ min}}$$

▶ **Answer:** 25 gtts/min

2. The patient is to receive 2000 cc of 5% dextrose and normal saline over 12 hours. The drop factor of the tubing is 15 gtts/cc. Determine the rate in gtts/min and in cc/h.

$$\frac{x \text{ gtts}}{\text{min}} = \frac{2000 \text{ cc}}{12 \text{ h}} \times \frac{15 \text{ gtts}}{1 \text{ cc}} \times \frac{1 \text{ h}}{60 \text{ min}}$$

$$\frac{x \text{ cc}}{\text{h}} = \frac{2000 \text{ cc}}{12 \text{ h}}$$

▶ **Answer:** 42 gtts/min and 167 cc/h

3. The physician has ordered 1000 cc of 5% dextrose alternating with 1000 cc of normal saline at a rate of 125 cc/h for the next 16 hours. The drop factor of the tubing is 20 gtts/cc. Determine the rate in gtts/min.

$$\frac{x \text{ gtts}}{\text{min}} = \frac{125 \text{ cc}}{1 \text{ h}} \times \frac{20 \text{ gtts}}{1 \text{ cc}} \times \frac{1 \text{ h}}{60 \text{ min}}$$

▶ **Answer:** 42 gtts/min

4. The order is to infuse 1500 cc of Ringer's lactate over the next 24 hours. The drop factor of the tubing is 60 gtts/cc. Determine the rate in gtts/min and cc/h.

$$\frac{x \text{ gtts}}{\text{min}} = \frac{1500 \text{ cc}}{24 \text{ h}} \times \frac{60 \text{ gtts}}{1 \text{ cc}} \times \frac{1 \text{ h}}{60 \text{ min}}$$

$$\frac{x \text{ cc}}{\text{h}} = \frac{1500 \text{ cc}}{24 \text{ h}}$$

▶ **Answer:** 63 gtts/min and 63 cc/h

5. The patient is to receive Intralipid 10% at a rate of 500 ml over 4 hours. The drop factor of the tubing is 10 gtts/cc. The product information states that the Intralipids should be administered at an initial rate of 1 cc/min for the first 15 to 30 minutes. Determine the initial rate and the rate for administration after the initial period. Express both answers in gtts/min.

$$\frac{x \text{ gtts}}{\text{min}} = \frac{1 \text{ cc}}{1 \text{ min}} \times \frac{10 \text{ gtts}}{\text{cc}} \quad \textit{Initial rate}$$

$$\frac{x \text{ gtts}}{\text{min}} = \frac{500 \text{ cc}}{4 \text{ h}} \times \frac{10 \text{ gtts}}{1 \text{ cc}} \times \frac{1 \text{ h}}{60 \text{ min}} \quad \textit{Final rate}$$

▶ **Answer:** Initial rate of 10 gtts/min, thereafter 21 gtts/min

▲ INFUSION OF BLOOD, BLOOD PRODUCTS, AND PLASMA EXPANDERS

Example 8.5: The order is to give 2 units of whole blood (1 unit is 500 cc). The blood is to infuse over the next 4 hours, and the drop factor of the tubing is 10 gtts/cc. Determine the rate in gtts/min required to transfuse as ordered.

Step 1: State the problem in equation form.

$$\frac{x \text{ gtts}}{\text{min}} = \frac{1000 \text{ cc}}{4 \text{ h}} \quad \text{Transfusing two 500 cc units}$$

Step 2: Identify the conversion factors needed to convert from cubic centimeters per hour to drops per minute.

Two conversion factors are used:

A. Convert from cubic centimeters to drops.

1 cc = 10 gtts

B. Convert from hours to minutes.

1 h = 60 min

Step 3: Put into the equation the form of each conversion factor that will cancel the unwanted labels and leave only the desired labels on both sides of the equal sign.

$$\frac{x \text{ gtts}}{\text{min}} = \frac{1000 \text{ cc}}{4 \text{ h}} \times \frac{10 \text{ gtts}}{1 \text{ cc}} \times \frac{1 \text{ h}}{60 \text{ min}}$$

Step 4: Cancel the labels that appear in both the numerator and the denominator on the same side of the equal sign.

$$\frac{x \text{ gtts}}{\text{min}} = \frac{1000}{4} \times \frac{10 \text{ gtts}}{1} \times \frac{1}{60 \text{ min}}$$

Step 5: Complete the required mathematical operations.

$$\frac{x \text{ gtts}}{\text{min}} = \frac{41.6 \text{ gtts}}{\text{min}}$$

Therefore, the rate is 42 gtts/min.

Example 8.6: The order is to give a stat dose of dextran 40, 500 ml over 90 minutes. The drop factor of the tubing is 12 gtts/ml. Determine the rate in gtts/min.

Step 1: State the problem in equation form.

$$\frac{x \text{ gtts}}{\text{min}} = \frac{500 \text{ ml}}{90 \text{ min}}$$

Step 2: Identify the conversion factor needed to convert from milliliters per minute to drops per minute: 12 gtts = 1 ml.

Step 3: Put into the equation the form of the conversion factor that will cancel the unwanted labels and leave only the desired labels on both sides of the equal sign.

$$\frac{x \text{ gtts}}{\text{min}} = \frac{500 \text{ ml}}{90 \text{ min}} \times \frac{12 \text{ gtts}}{1 \text{ ml}}$$

Step 4: Cancel the labels that appear in both the numerator and the denominator on the same side of the equal sign.

$$\frac{x \text{ gtts}}{\text{min}} = \frac{500}{90 \text{ min}} \times \frac{12 \text{ gtts}}{1}$$

Step 5: Complete the required mathematical operations.

$$\frac{x \text{ gtts}}{\text{min}} = \frac{66.7 \text{ gtts}}{\text{min}}$$

Therefore, the rate is 67 gtts/min.

Example 8.7: The physician has ordered 50 cc of 5% normal albumin to be given over 15 minutes. The drop factor of the tubing is 10 gtts/cc. Determine the rate in gtts/min.

Step 1: State the problem in equation form.

$$\frac{x \text{ gtts}}{\text{min}} = \frac{50 \text{ cc}}{15 \text{ min}}$$

Step 2: Identify the conversion factor needed to convert from cubic centimeters per minute to drops per minute: 10 gtts = 1 cc.

Step 3: Put into the equation the form of the conversion factor that will cancel the unwanted labels and leave only the desired labels on both sides of the equal sign.

$$\frac{x \text{ gtts}}{\text{min}} = \frac{50 \text{ cc}}{15 \text{ min}} \times \frac{10 \text{ gtts}}{1 \text{ cc}}$$

Step 4: Cancel the labels that appear in both the numerator and the denominator on the same side of the equal sign.

$$\frac{x \text{ gtts}}{\text{min}} = \frac{50}{15 \text{ min}} \times \frac{10 \text{ gtts}}{1}$$

Step 5: Complete the required mathematical operations.

$$\frac{x \text{ gtts}}{\text{min}} = \frac{33.3 \text{ gtts}}{\text{min}}$$

Therefore, the rate is 33 gtts/min.

► SOLVED PRACTICE PROBLEMS

1. The patient is to receive 3 units of whole blood. Each unit contains 500 cc. The blood is to be infused over the next 6 hours. The drop factor of the tubing is 10 gtts/cc. Determine the rate in gtts/min.

$$\frac{x \text{ gtts}}{\text{min}} = \frac{1500 \text{ cc}}{6 \text{ h}} \times \frac{10 \text{ gtts}}{1 \text{ cc}} \times \frac{1 \text{ h}}{60 \text{ min}}$$

► **Answer:** 42 gtts/min

2. The patient is to receive a transfusion of washed, packed red blood cells. Three units of 250 cc each are ordered to be infused in 4 hours. The drop factor of the tubing is 12 gtts/cc. Determine the rate of gtts/min.

$$\frac{x \text{ gtts}}{\text{min}} = \frac{750 \text{ cc}}{4 \text{ h}} \times \frac{12 \text{ gtts}}{1 \text{ cc}} \times \frac{1 \text{ h}}{60 \text{ min}}$$

▶ **Answer:** 38 gtts/min

3. The order is to give 250 ml of Rheomacrodex (dextran 40) over 45 minutes. The drop factor of the tubing is 10 gtts/cc. Determine the rate in gtts/min.

$$\frac{x \text{ gtts}}{\text{min}} = \frac{250 \text{ ml}}{45 \text{ min}} \times \frac{10 \text{ gtts}}{1 \text{ ml}}$$

▶ **Answer:** 56 gtts/min

4. The order is to infuse Plasmanate (plasma protein fraction) at a rate of 4 ml per minute for a total dose of 500 ml. The drop factor of the tubing is 10 gtts/ml. Determine the rate in gtts/min.

$$\frac{x \text{ gtts}}{\text{min}} = \frac{4 \text{ ml}}{1 \text{ min}} \times \frac{10 \text{ gtts}}{1 \text{ ml}}$$

▶ **Answer:** 40 gtts/min

5. The order is to give plasma protein fraction, 8 ml/min up to a total dose of 250 ml. The drop factor of the tubing is 12 gtts/cc. Determine the rate in gtts/min.

$$\frac{x \text{ gtts}}{\text{min}} = \frac{8 \text{ ml}}{1 \text{ min}} \times \frac{12 \text{ gtts}}{1 \text{ ml}}$$

▶ **Answer:** 96 gtts/min

▲ ADDITION OF KCl TO IV FLUIDS

Potassium chloride (KCl) is a common additive in IV fluids. KCl is supplied in a solution with a concentration of 2 mEq per ml. When added to small amounts of IV fluid, the volume of the KCl is usually included in the calculation of the infusion rate. For example, if 20 ml of KCl (40 mEq) are added to 100 ml of IV fluid, the infusion rate would be calculated for a total of 120 ml (100 ml IV + 20 ml KCl) of fluid. This is illustrated in Example 8.8.

Frequently, physicians change the number of mEq of KCl to be added to a liter of IV fluid. Whenever the number of mEq is increased, it is possible to add the needed amount of KCl to the remaining IV fluid. Since IV fluids are expensive, where policy permits, nurses should add the required KCl rather than discard large amounts of IV fluid. The method used to determine the number of mEq of KCl to be added to the remaining solution is described in Examples 8.9 and 8.10.

Example 8.8: The physician has ordered 60 mEq to be added to 100 cc of 5% dextrose to run in over 6 hours. The KCl is supplied in multiple-dose vials of 2 mEq per cc. Determine the rate of the IV using a drop factor of 60 gtts/cc.

First calculate the volume of KCl to be added to the 100 cc of IV fluid.

Step 1: State the problem in equation form.

$$x \text{ cc} = 60 \text{ mEq}$$

Step 2: Identify the conversion factor needed to convert from mEq to cubic centimeters: 1 cc = 2 mEq.

Step 3: Put into the equation the form of the conversion factor that will cancel the unwanted label and leave only the desired label on both sides of the equal sign.

$$x \text{ cc} = 60 \text{ mEq} \times \frac{1 \text{ cc}}{2 \text{ mEq}}$$

Step 4: Cancel the labels that appear in both the numerator and the denominator on the same side of the equal sign.

$$x \text{ cc} = 60 \times \frac{1 \text{ cc}}{2}$$

Step 5: Complete the required mathematical operations.

$$x \text{ cc} = 30 \text{ cc}$$

Therefore, the total amount of fluid to be infused is 100 cc + 30 cc = 130 cc. The IV rate must be calculated to administer 130 cc (not 100 cc) over 6 hours.

Step 1: State the problem in equation form.

$$\frac{x \text{ gtts}}{\text{min}} = \frac{130 \text{ cc}}{6 \text{ h}}$$

Step 2: Identify the conversion factors needed to convert from cubic centimeters per hour to drops per minute.

Two conversion factors are used:

A. Convert from cubic centimeters to drops.

1 cc = 60 gtts

B. Convert from hours to minutes.

1 h = 60 min

Step 3: Put into the equation the form of each conversion factor that will cancel the unwanted labels and leave only the desired labels on both sides of the equal sign.

$$\frac{x \text{ gtts}}{\text{min}} = \frac{130 \text{ cc}}{6 \text{ h}} \times \frac{60 \text{ gtts}}{1 \text{ cc}} \times \frac{1 \text{ h}}{60 \text{ min}}$$

Step 4: Cancel the labels that appear in both the numerator and the denominator on the same side of the equal sign.

$$\frac{x \text{ gtts}}{\text{min}} = \frac{130}{6} \times \frac{60 \text{ gtts}}{1} \times \frac{1}{60 \text{ min}}$$

Step 5: Complete the required mathematical operations.

$$\frac{x \text{ gtts}}{\text{min}} = \frac{21.6 \text{ gtts}}{\text{min}}$$

Therefore, the rate is 22 gtts/min.

In general, when liquid forms of medication are added to IV fluids, it is a safe practice to include the added volume in the calculation of the IV rate.

Example 8.9: An IV of 1000 ml of 5% dextrose with 10 mEq of KCl is infusing with 500 ml remaining in the bag. The new orders are to increase the KCl to 20 mEq per 1000 ml. If the decision is made not to discard the current IV, but to increase the KCl to the ordered concentration, how many mEq of KCl should be added to the remaining 500 ml?

The problem is solved in three steps as indicated below. These steps are illustrated in Figure 8–3.

1. Determine the *desired* number of mEq of KCl in the *remaining* IV solution.

   $x \text{ mEq} = 500 \text{ ml}$

   Conversion factor needed: 1000 ml = 20 mEq (new order)

   $$x \text{ mEq} = 500 \text{ ml} \times \frac{20 \text{ mEq}}{1000 \text{ ml}}$$

   $$x \text{ mEq} = 500 \times \frac{20 \text{ mEq}}{1000}$$

   $x \text{ mEq} = 10 \text{ mEq}$

2. Determine the *current* number of mEq of KCl in the *remaining* IV solution.

   $x \text{ mEq} = 500 \text{ ml}$

   Conversion factor needed: 1000 ml = 10 mEq (original order).

   $$x \text{ mEq} = 500 \text{ ml} \times \frac{10 \text{ mEq}}{1000 \text{ ml}}$$

   $$x \text{ mEq} = 500 \times \frac{10 \text{ mEq}}{1000}$$

   $x \text{ mEq} = 5 \text{ mEq}$

3. Determine the number of mEq to be added to the remaining solution. mEq to be added = desired mEq − current mEq.

   $5 \text{ mEq} = 10 \text{ mEq} - 5 \text{ mEq}$

   Therefore, add 5 mEq to the remaining 500 ml of IV.

   Refer to the label for KCl in Figure 8–3. How many ml would be needed to equal 5 mEq of KCl?

   Answer:

   $$x \text{ ml} = 5 \text{ mEq} \times \frac{30 \text{ ml}}{60 \text{ mEq}}$$

   $x \text{ ml} = 2.5 \text{ ml}$

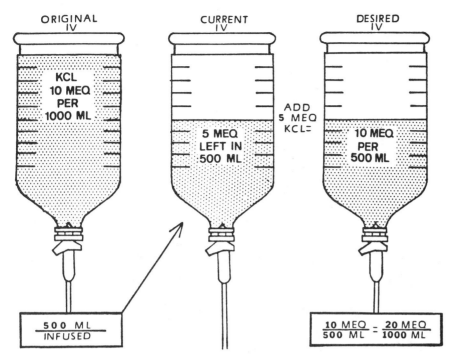

Increasing the mEq of KCl in IV fluid.

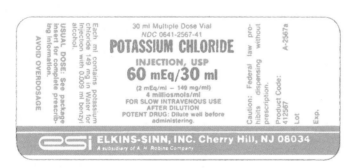

FIGURE 8-3.

Example 8.10: The order is to infuse 1000 cc of 5% dextrose with 40 mEq KCl at 100 cc/h. Presently infusing is 1000 cc of 5% dextrose with 800 cc of fluid remaining to be infused. How many mEq of KCl should you add to the present bag to bring it to the desired concentration?

1. Determine the *desired* number of mEq of KCl in the *remaining* IV solution.

x mEq = 800 cc

Conversion factor needed: 1000 cc = 40 mEq (new order).

$$x \text{ mEq} = 800 \text{ cc} \times \frac{40 \text{ mEq}}{1000 \text{ cc}}$$

$$x \text{ mEq} = 800 \times \frac{40 \text{ mEq}}{1000}$$

$$x \text{ mEq} = 32 \text{ mEq}$$

2. Determine the *current* number of mEq of KCl in the *remaining* IV solution.

x mEq $=$ 800 cc

Conversion factor needed: 1000 cc $=$ 0 mEq (original order). There is *no* mEq of KCl in the original order.

$$x \text{ mEq} = 800 \text{ cc} \times \frac{0 \text{ mEq}}{1000 \text{ cc}}$$

$$x \text{ mEq} = 800 \times \frac{0 \text{ mEq}}{1000}$$

$$x \text{ mEq} = 0 \text{ mEq}$$

3. Determine the number of mEq to be added to the remaining IV solution. mEq to be added $=$ desired mEq $-$ current mEq.

32 mEq $=$ 32 mEq $-$ 0 mEq

Therefore, add 24 mEq to the remaining 800 cc of IV.

► SOLVED PRACTICE PROBLEMS

1. The physician orders an IV of 1000 cc of 5% dextrose and normal saline to have 20 mEq of KCl added. The KCl is available in multiple dose vials with 2 mEq per cc. How many cc of KCl should be added to the IV solution?

$$x \text{ cc} = 20 \text{ mEq} \times \frac{1 \text{ cc}}{2 \text{ mEq}}$$

► **Answer:** 10 cc

2. An IV of 1000 cc of 5% dextrose with 10 mEq of KCl has 700 cc to be absorbed. The order is to increase the KCl to 30 mEq per liter. How many mEq will you add to the present IV?

Desired mEq KCl $= 700 \text{ cc} \times \dfrac{30 \text{ mEq}}{1000 \text{ cc}}$ Desired $= 21$ mEq

Current mEq KCl $= 700 \text{ cc} \times \dfrac{10 \text{ mEq}}{1000 \text{ cc}}$ Current $= 7$ mEq

mEq to be added $= 21 \text{ mEq} - 7 \text{ mEq}$ Add   14 mEq

► **Answer:** 14 mEq

3. The order is to add 40 mEq of KCl to 80 cc of 5% dextrose and infuse over 4 hours. The drop factor of the tubing is 60 gtts/cc. Determine the rate in gtts/min. The KCl is supplied 2 mEq per cc.

$$\frac{x \text{ gtts}}{\text{min}} = \frac{100 \text{ cc}}{4 \text{ h}} \times \frac{60 \text{ gtts}}{1 \text{ cc}} \times \frac{1 \text{ h}}{60 \text{ min}}$$

The calculated rate is based on the addition of 20 cc of KCl (40 mEq) to 80 cc of 5% dextrose solution to give a total IV volume of 100 cc.

► **Answer:** 25 gtts/min

4. An IV of Ringer's lactate with 10 mEq of KCl has 700 cc remaining. The order is to increase the KCl from 10 mEq per liter to 40 mEq per liter. How many mEq of KCl will you add to the remaining 700 cc?

$$\text{Desired mEq KCl} = 700 \text{ cc} \times \frac{40 \text{ mEq}}{1000 \text{ cc}} \qquad \text{Desired} = 28 \text{ mEq}$$

$$\text{Current mEq KCl} = 700 \text{ cc} \times \frac{10 \text{ mEq}}{1000 \text{ cc}} \qquad \text{Current} = 7 \text{ mEq}$$

$$\text{mEq to be added} = 28 \text{ mEq} - 7 \text{ mEq} \qquad \text{Add} \qquad 21 \text{ mEq}$$

▶ **Answer:** 21 mEq KCl

5. An IV of 500 cc of 5% dextrose with 20 mEq of KCl has 400 cc remaining. A new order has been written for 1000 cc of 5% dextrose with 40 mEq KCl. How many mEq of KCl should be added to the present IV?

$$\text{Desired mEq KCl} = 400 \text{ cc} \times \frac{40 \text{ mEq}}{1000 \text{ cc}} \qquad \text{Desired} = 16 \text{ mEq}$$

$$\text{Current mEq KCl} = 400 \text{ cc} \times \frac{20 \text{ mEq}}{500 \text{ cc}} \qquad \text{Current} = 16 \text{ mEq}$$

$$\text{mEq to be added} = 16 \text{ mEq} - 16 \text{ mEq} \qquad \text{Add} \qquad 0 \text{ mEq}$$

▶ **Answer:** No additional KCl needs to be added

CASE STUDY

▶ Case Eight

R.K., a 23-year-old female, has been admitted with a diagnosis of dehydration. She has a history of ulcerative colitis and experienced severe diarrhea for several days prior to admission. Her original IV order upon admission was: 1000 cc 5% dextrose and 0.45% sodium chloride with 20 mEq KCl (D_5W ½ NS with 20 mEq KCl) to run at a 6-hour rate. A new order has been written to slow the IV to an 8 hour rate and change the KCl to 30 mEq/L. The current IV of D_5W ½ NS with 20 mEq KCl has 800 cc remaining to be absorbed. The IV infusion set being used delivers 15 gtts/cc.

1. With the original IV order, how many cc of IV fluid was the patient receiving in 24 hours?
2. What rate (gtts/min) was needed to administer 1000 cc of IV fluid over a 6-hour period?
3. With the new IV order, how many cc of IV fluid will the patient now receive in 24 hours?
4. What rate (cc/h) is now needed to administer 1000 cc of IV fluid over an 8-hour period?
5. What rate (gtts/min) is now needed to administer 1000 cc of IV fluid over an 8-hour period?
6. How many mEq of KCl were present in 1000 cc of the original IV?
7. How many mEq of KCl would be present in 1000 cc of the new IV?
8. How many mEq of KCl are present in the remaining 800 cc of the original IV?

9. How many mEq of KCl should be present in 800 cc of the new IV?
10. How many mEq of KCl should be added to the 800 cc of D_5W ½ NS with 20 mEq KCl to increase the KCl as ordered?

For answers to Case Study Eight, see page 155.

▶ SELF-TEST

1. The order is to give 1000 cc of 5% dextrose and 0.45% sodium chloride over 6 hours. Using a drop factor of 10 gtts/cc, find the rate in gtts/min and in cc/h.
2. The physician has ordered 1000 cc of 5% dextrose to alternate with 1000 cc 0.45% sodium chloride over the next 24 hours at a rate of 150 cc/h. Using 15 gtts/cc, determine the rate in gtts/min.
3. The order is for Ringer's lactate 500 cc q8h. Using 60 gtts/cc, determine the gtts/min and cc/h needed.
4. The order is to infuse 1000 cc of 5% dextrose over 24 hours to keep the vein open. Using 60 gtts/cc, determine the rate in gtts/min and cc/h.
5. The physician has ordered two units of whole blood (500 cc each) over the next 5 hours. Using 10 gtts/cc, determine the rate in gtts/min.
6. The physician has ordered 250 ml of dextran 40 to be given over the next 90 minutes. The drop factor is 12 gtts/cc. Find the rate in gtts/min.
7. The order is to infuse two units of washed, packed red cells (250 cc each) over the next 3 hours. Using a drop factor of 10 gtts/cc, find the rate in gtts/min.
8. The patient is to receive 3 liters of 5% dextrose in 0.45% sodium chloride over the next 24 hours. The drop factor is 10 gtts/cc. Determine the rate of the IV in gtts/min.
9. The patient is to receive 3 units of whole blood (1 unit is approximately 500 cc) over the next 6 hours. The drop factor of the tubing is 10 gtts/cc. Determine the rate of the infusion in gtts/min.
10. The order is to give 250 ml of dextran 40 over 60 minutes. The drop factor of the tubing is 10 gtts/cc. Determine the rate of the infusion in gtts/min.
11. The order is to infuse 1000 cc of 5% dextrose and normal saline with 40 mEq of KCl. Currently infusing is 1000 cc of 5% dextrose and normal saline with 20 mEq of KCl with 900 cc remaining. How many mEq of KCl should you add to the present bag to bring the KCl to the desired concentration?
12. The order is to add 30 mEq of KCl to 1000 cc of 5% dextrose and 0.45% sodium chloride. The KCl is supplied in an ampule with 40 mEq per 20 cc. How many cc of KCl will you add to the IV?
13. The physician has ordered 50 mEq of KCl to be added to 100 cc of IV fluid and administered at a rate of 10 mEq per hour for the next

Continued next page

▶ **Self-Test Continued**

5 hours. KCl is supplied in multiple-dose vials in a concentration of 2 mEq per 1 cc. Using 60 gtts/cc, find the rate in gtts/min.

14. The IV in progress is 1000 cc of normal saline with 10 mEq of KCl, and 800 cc remain to be absorbed. The order is to increase the KCl to 40 mEq per liter. How many mEq of KCl will you add to the 800 cc remaining?

15. The order is to add 30 mEq per liter to the 5% dextrose IV solution. There are 600 cc remaining of the 1000 cc IV of the 5% dextrose. How many cc of KCl will you add if the KCl is supplied 2 mEq per 1 cc?

For answers to the self-test, see below.

1. 4000 cc	5. 31 gtts/min	8. 16 mEq
2. 42 gtts/min	6. 20 mEq	9. 24 mEq
3. 3000 cc	7. 30 mEq	10. 8 mEq
4. 125 cc/h		

1. 28 gtts/min and 167 cc/h	6. 33 gtts/min	11. 18 mEq
2. 38 gtts/min	7. 28 gtts/min	12. 15 cc
3. 63 gtts/min and 63 cc/h	8. 21 gtts/min	13. 25 gtts/min
4. 42 gtts/min and 42 cc/h	9. 42 gtts/min	14. 24 mEq
5. 33 gtts/min	10. 42 gtts/min	15. 9 cc

ANSWERS to Case Study Eight

ANSWERS to Self-test

Intravenous Medications

9

▲ OBJECTIVES

Upon completion of Chapter 9, the student will be able to:

- ▶ Consistently express the rate of an IV infusion, calculated in either drops per minute or milliliters per hour, in whole numbers only.

- ▶ Correctly calculate the rate in drops per minute or in milliliters per hour for IV medications given by intermittent infusion given:
  Any drop factor
  The recommended dilution
  The recommended time period for administration

- ▶ Correctly calculate the rate in drops per minute or in milliliters per hour for IV medications given by continuous infusion given:
  Any drop factor
  The time period for administration
  The amount of medication in the IV

- ▶ Correctly calculate the dosage (e.g., mg/min) for IV medications given by continuous infusion given:
  The amount of medication in the IV
  The rate in milliliters per hour

▲ INTRODUCTION TO ADMINISTRATION OF INTRAVENOUS MEDICATIONS

Intravenous medications may be given by continuous or intermittent infusion. For medications given by intermittent infusion, the physician usually indicates the type and amount of medication to be given at specific intervals, relying on the nurse to follow the manufacturer's recommendations for dilution and rate of administration.

Intermittent infusion requires giving a drug through an in-progress IV or through a special intravenous catheter (such as a heparin lock) adapted to periodic administration of medications. Intermittent infusion of IV medications can be accomplished through the use of the following:

1. Volume control set: Allows the medication to be injected into a specific volume of compatible IV fluid and then administered in minidrops over

a specific period of time (dilution and rate varying with the manufacturer's recommendations)

2. Secondary line: Addition of second container with medication and compatible IV fluid to an in-progress IV or to a heparin lock; flow rate is adjusted for administration of the diluted medication

The terms *piggyback* and *intravenous piggyback* (IVPB) are commonly used when referring to any intermittent administration of medication that requires more than 5 minutes to complete; usually 20–30 minutes is required for infusing the diluted medication. The terms *push* and *IV push* (IVP) are commonly used when referring to any intravenous medication injected in 5 minutes or less.

If medications are to be given by continuous infusion, the physician will specify the amount of medication to be added to a certain volume of IV fluid. The medication is then administered in the IV fluid, requiring the same amount of time to infuse as the IV fluid.

For medications given by continuous infusion, the physician may order the rate of infusion in terms other than milliliters per hour. For example, the order may specify a certain number of milligrams per hour, units per hour, or micrograms per minute. Table 9–1 indicates medications that are commonly ordered in this fashion.

▶ alert:

When certain IV medications are infused at an incorrect rate, serious adverse reactions can occur.

▶ critical decision point:

The order reads: *Continuous IV of 1200 units of heparin per hour.* You are told at change-of-shift that a new 1000 cc IV bag with 30,000 units of heparin was hung at 6 AM. It is now 4 PM and you are making rounds. You note that there are 200 cc of IV solution remaining in the bag. You determine from the time tape on the bag that there should be 600 cc remaining at this time. You realize that 400 cc more of IV fluid have been infused than should have been by this point.

▶ decision/action:

You realize that since 1000 cc of IV fluid contain 30,000 units of heparin, each 100 cc contain 3000 units. You know that the 400 cc of extra IV infused contained 12,000 units of heparin. You recognize that your BEST action now is to stop the IV and notify the physician, who will probably order the IV continue to be held until appropriate lab results can be obtained.

TABLE 9–1. MEDICATIONS ADMINISTERED BY CONTINUOUS INFUSION

Medication	Rate of Infusion Expressed as	
Isoproterenol	Micrograms per minute	(mcg/min)
Lidocaine	Milligrams per minute	(mg/min)
Morphine	Milligrams per minute	(mg/min)
Ritodrine	Milligrams per minute	(mg/min)
Oxytocin	Milliunits per minute	(mU/min)
Aminophylline	Milligrams per hour	(mg/hr)
Heparin	Units per hour	(U/hr)

▲ INTERMITTENT INFUSION OF MEDICATIONS

Infusion rates for medications administered intermittently (IVPB) are calculated according to the method illustrated in Chapter 8. Frequently the nurse must determine the proper dilution and rate of administration of the medication based on the manufacturer's recommendation. Often the manufacturer recommends a range of dilutions and a range of infusion times. For example, a given medication may have a recommended dilution of 50–100 ml of compatible IV fluid and a recommended infusion time of 15–30 minutes. The nurse selects both a dilution and an infusion time appropriate to the patient.

Example 9.1: The order is to give Tagamet (cimetidine) 300 mg IVPB q6h. It is recommended that this medication be dissolved in 50–100 cc of compatible IV solution and infused over 15–30 minutes. Using a drop factor of 20 gtts/cc, determine the rate needed to infuse the Tagamet in 100 cc over 30 minutes.

Step 1:   State the problem in equation form.

$$\frac{x \text{ gtts}}{\text{min}} = \frac{100 \text{ cc}}{30 \text{ min}}$$

Step 2:   Identify the conversion factor needed to convert from cubic centimeters per minute to drops per minute: 20 gtts = 1 cc.

Step 3:   Put into the equation the form of the conversion factor that will cancel the unwanted labels and leave only the desired labels on both sides of the equal sign.

$$\frac{x \text{ gtts}}{\text{min}} = \frac{100 \text{ cc}}{30 \text{ min}} \times \frac{20 \text{ gtts}}{1 \text{ cc}}$$

Step 4:   Cancel the labels that appear in both the numerator and the denominator on the same side of the equal sign.

$$\frac{x \text{ gtts}}{\text{min}} = \frac{100}{30 \text{ min}} \times \frac{20 \text{ gtts}}{1}$$

Step 5:   Complete the required mathematical operations.

$$\frac{x \text{ gtts}}{\text{min}} = \frac{66.7 \text{ gtts}}{\text{min}}$$

Therefore, the rate is 67 gtts/min.

Example 9.2: The order is to give 6 million units of penicillin G q4h, IVPB. The medication is to be dissolved in 150 cc of IV fluid and the recommended infusion time is 1½ hours. Using a drop factor of 10 gtts/cc, determine the rate in gtts/min.

Step 1:   State the problem in equation form.

$$\frac{x \text{ gtts}}{\text{min}} = \frac{150 \text{ cc}}{1.5 \text{ h}}$$

Step 2:   Identify the conversion factors needed to convert from cubic centimeters per hour to drops per minute.

Two conversion factors are used:

A. Convert from cubic centimeters to drops.

$$1 \text{ cc } = 10 \text{ gtts}$$

B. Convert from hours to minutes.

$$1 \text{ h } = 60 \text{ min}$$

Step 3: Put into the equation the form of each conversion factor that will cancel the unwanted labels and leave only the desired labels on both sides of the equal sign.

$$\frac{x \text{ gtts}}{\text{min}} = \frac{150 \text{ cc}}{1.5 \text{ h}} \times \frac{10 \text{ gtts}}{1 \text{ cc}} \times \frac{1 \text{ h}}{60 \text{ min}}$$

Step 4: Cancel the labels that appear in both the numerator and the denominator on the same side of the equal sign.

$$\frac{x \text{ gtts}}{\text{min}} = \frac{150}{1.5} \times \frac{10 \text{ gtts}}{1} \times \frac{1}{60 \text{ min}}$$

Step 5: Complete the required mathematical operations.

$$\frac{x \text{ gtts}}{\text{min}} = \frac{16.7 \text{ gtts}}{\text{min}}$$

Therefore, the rate is 17 gtts/min.

► SOLVED PRACTICE PROBLEMS

1. The order is to give Unipen (nafcillin) 500 mg IVPB q6h. The recommended dilution is 500 mg in 50 ml of IV solution to be administered over 15–30 minutes. Using a drop factor of 10 gtts/cc, determine the rate needed to infuse the medication in 15 minutes.

$$\frac{x \text{ gtts}}{\text{min}} = \frac{50 \text{ ml}}{15 \text{ min}} \times \frac{10 \text{ gtts}}{1 \text{ ml}}$$

► **Answer:** 33 gtts/min

2. The patient is to receive Aldomet (methyldopa) 500 mg IVPB. The medication is dissolved in 100 cc of IV fluid. Each 500 mg is to be run in over 1 hour. Using a drop factor of 15 gtts/cc, determine the rate in gtts/min.

$$\frac{x \text{ gtts}}{\text{min}} = \frac{100 \text{ cc}}{1 \text{ h}} \times \frac{15 \text{ gtts}}{1 \text{ cc}} \times \frac{1 \text{ h}}{60 \text{ min}}$$

► **Answer:** 25 gtts/min

3. The order is to give 100 mg of Aminophylline (theophylline) in a total of 35 cc of fluid over the next 45 minutes. Using a drop factor of 60 gtts/cc, determine the rate of gtts/min.

$$\frac{x \text{ gtts}}{\text{min}} = \frac{35 \text{ cc}}{45 \text{ min}} \times \frac{60 \text{ gtts}}{1 \text{ cc}}$$

► **Answer:** 47 gtts/min

4. The order is to give Keflin (cephalothin) 2 g q6h IVPB. The recommended dilution is 50 ml of IV fluid. The medication may be given over 15–30 minutes. Using a drop factor of 60 gtts/cc, determine the rate for administration over 30 minutes.

$$\frac{x \text{ gtts}}{\text{min}} = \frac{50 \text{ ml}}{30 \text{ min}} \times \frac{60 \text{ gtts}}{1 \text{ ml}}$$

► **Answer:** 100 gtts/min

5. The order is to give 80 mg of tobramycin q4h IVPB. The medication is dissolved in 100 cc of IV fluid and recommended rate of administration is 30–60 minutes. Using a drop factor of 10 gtts/cc, determine the rate for administration over 60 minutes.

$$\frac{x \text{ gtts}}{\text{min}} = \frac{100 \text{ cc}}{60 \text{ min}} \times \frac{10 \text{ gtts}}{1 \text{ cc}}$$

► **Answer:** 17 gtts/min

▲ CONTINUOUS INFUSION OF MEDICATIONS

Infusion rates for medications administered continuously are calculated according to the manner in which the physician orders the medication. When the rate of infusion is ordered in terms specified in Table 9–1 (e.g., mg/h, μg/min) the method of calculation used must include both the specified rate of infusion and the concentration of the medication in the IV solution.

When calculating infusion rates ordered in terms such as milligrams per minute, the following are considered to be conversion factors:

1. The drop factor of the infusion set (used only when rate is calculated in drops per minute)
2. The concentration of the medication in the IV solution, usually expressed as the number of milligrams or units of medication in the total solution (e.g., 30,000 units per 1000 ml)

Calculation of Rate in Drops Per Minute or Cubic Centimeters Per Hour

Example 9.3: The order is to give 1200 units of heparin per hour; the directions for the IV are to add 30,000 units of heparin to each 1000 cc of solution. Using tubing with a drop factor of 60 gtts/cc, determine the rate in gtts/min and cc/h.

Part 1: Find Drops per Minute

Step 1: State the problem in equation form.

$$\frac{x \text{ gtts}}{\text{min}} = \frac{1200 \text{ U}}{1 \text{ h}}$$

Step 2: Identify the conversion factors needed to convert from units per hour to drops per minute. The information needed from the problem to identify the conversion factors is: There are 60 gtts per cc; there are 30,000 units per 1000 cc of IV fluid.

Three conversion factors are used:

A. Convert from units to cubic centimeters.

30,000 U = 1000 cc

B. Convert from cubic centimeters to drops.

1 cc = 60 gtts

C. Convert from hours to minutes.

1 h = 60 min

Step 3: Put into the equation the form of each conversion factor that will cancel the unwanted labels and leave only the desired labels on both sides of the equal sign.

$$\frac{x \text{ gtts}}{\text{min}} = \frac{1200 \text{ U}}{1 \text{ h}} \times \frac{1000 \text{ cc}}{30,000 \text{ U}} \times \frac{60 \text{ gtts}}{1 \text{ cc}} \times \frac{1 \text{ h}}{60 \text{ min}}$$

Step 4: Cancel the labels that appear in both the numerator and the denominator on the same side of the equal sign.

$$\frac{x \text{ gtts}}{\text{min}} = \frac{1200}{1} \times \frac{1000}{30,000} \times \frac{60 \text{ gtts}}{1} \times \frac{1}{60 \text{ min}}$$

Step 5: Complete the required mathematical operations.

$$\frac{x \text{ gtts}}{\text{min}} = \frac{40 \text{ gtts}}{\text{min}}$$

Therefore, the rate is 40 gtts/min.

Part 2: Find Cubic Centimeters per Hour

Step 1: State the problem in equation form.

$$\frac{x \text{ cc}}{\text{h}} = \frac{1200 \text{ U}}{1 \text{ h}}$$

Step 2: Identify the conversion factor needed to convert from units per hour to cubic centimeters per hour. The information needed from the problem to identify the conversion factor is: There are 30,000 units per 1000 cc of IV fluid (30,000 U = 1000 cc).

Step 3: Put into the equation the form of the conversion factor that will cancel the unwanted labels and leave only the desired labels on both sides of the equal sign.

$$\frac{x \text{ cc}}{\text{h}} = \frac{1200 \text{ U}}{1 \text{ h}} \times \frac{1000 \text{ cc}}{30,000 \text{ U}}$$

Step 4: Cancel the labels that appear in both the numerator and the denominator on the same side of the equal sign.

$$\frac{x \text{ cc}}{\text{h}} = \frac{1200}{\text{h}} \times \frac{1000 \text{ cc}}{30,000}$$

Step 5: Complete the required mathematical operations.

$$\frac{x \text{ cc}}{\text{h}} = \frac{40 \text{ cc}}{\text{h}}$$

Therefore, the rate is 40 cc/h.

Example 9.4: The physician has ordered a continuous infusion of theophylline at a rate of 25 mg per hour. The theophylline is mixed in 5% dextrose to produce a concentration of 500 mg per 500 cc. Using a drop factor of 20 gtts/cc, determine the rate of the IV in gtts/min.

Step 1: State the problem in equation form:

$$\frac{x \text{ gtts}}{\text{min}} = \frac{25 \text{ mg}}{\text{h}}$$

Step 2: Identify the conversion factors needed to convert from milligrams per hour to drops per minute. The information needed from the problem to identify the conversion factors is: There are 20 gtts per cc; there are 500 mg per 500 cc of IV fluid.

Three conversion factors are used:

A. Convert from milligrams to cubic centimeters.

$$500 \text{ mg} = 500 \text{ cc}$$

B. Convert from cubic centimeters to drops.

$$1 \text{ cc} = 20 \text{ gtts}$$

C. Convert from hours to minutes.

$$1 \text{ h} = 60 \text{ min}$$

Step 3: Put into the equation the form of each conversion factor that will cancel the unwanted labels and leave only the desired labels on both sides of the equal sign.

$$\frac{x \text{ gtts}}{\text{min}} = \frac{25 \text{ mg}}{1 \text{ h}} \times \frac{500 \text{ cc}}{500 \text{ mg}} \times \frac{20 \text{ gtts}}{1 \text{ cc}} \times \frac{1 \text{ h}}{60 \text{ min}}$$

Step 4: Cancel the labels that appear in both the numerator and the denominator on the same side of the equal sign.

$$\frac{x \text{ gtts}}{\text{min}} = \frac{25}{1} \times \frac{500}{500} \times \frac{20 \text{ gtts}}{1} \times \frac{1}{60 \text{ min}}$$

Step 5: Complete the required mathematical operations.

$$\frac{x \text{ gtts}}{\text{min}} = \frac{8.3 \text{ gtts}}{\text{min}}$$

Therefore, the rate is 8 gtts/min.

Example 9.5: The patient is to receive 8 milliunits (mU) per minute of Pitocin (oxytocin). The directions are to add 10 units of Pitocin to 1 liter (L) of 5% dextrose solution. Determine the rate of the IV in gtts/min and cc/h using a drop factor of 60 gtts/cc.

Part 1: Find Drops per Minute

Step 1: State the problem in equation form.

$$\frac{x \text{ gtts}}{\text{min}} = \frac{8 \text{ mU}}{1 \text{ min}}$$

Step 2: Identify the conversion factors needed to convert from milliunits per minute to drops per minute. The information needed from the problem to identify the conversion factors is: There are 60 drops per cc; there are 10 units per 1000 cc IV fluid.

Three conversion factors are used:

A. Convert from milliunits to units

$$1000 \, \text{mU} = 1 \, \text{U}$$

B. Convert from units to cubic centimeters.

$$10 \, \text{U} = 1000 \, \text{cc}$$

C. Convert from cubic centimeters to drops.

$$1 \, \text{cc} = 60 \, \text{gtts}$$

Step 3: Put into the equation the form of each conversion factor that will cancel the unwanted labels and leave only the desired labels on both sides of the equal sign.

$$\frac{x \, \text{gtts}}{\text{min}} = \frac{8 \, \text{mU}}{1 \, \text{min}} \times \frac{1 \, \text{U}}{1000 \, \text{mU}} \times \frac{1000 \, \text{cc}}{10 \, \text{U}} \times \frac{60 \, \text{gtts}}{1 \, \text{cc}}$$

Step 4: Cancel the labels that appear in both the numerator and the denominator on the same side of the equal sign.

$$\frac{x \, \text{gtts}}{\text{min}} = \frac{8}{1 \, \text{min}} \times \frac{1}{1000} \times \frac{1000}{10} \times \frac{60 \, \text{gtts}}{1}$$

Step 5: Complete the required mathematical operations.

$$\frac{x \, \text{gtts}}{\text{min}} = \frac{48 \, \text{gtts}}{\text{min}}$$

Therefore, the rate is 48 gtts/min.

Part 2: Find Cubic Centimeters per Hour

Step 1: State the problem in equation form.

$$\frac{x \, \text{cc}}{\text{h}} = \frac{8 \, \text{mU}}{1 \, \text{min}}$$

Step 2: Identify the conversion factors needed to convert from milliunits per minute to cubic centimeters per hour. The information needed from the problem to identify the conversion factors is: There are 10 units per 1000 cc of IV fluid.

Three conversion factors are used:

A. Convert from milliunits to units.

$$1000 \, \text{mU} = 1 \, \text{U}$$

B. Convert from units to cubic centimeters.

$$10 \, \text{U} = 1000 \, \text{cc}$$

C. Convert from minutes to hours.

$$60 \, \text{min} = 1 \, \text{h}$$

Step 3: Put into the equation the form of each conversion factor that will cancel the unwanted labels and leave only the desired labels on both sides of the equal sign.

$$\frac{x \text{ cc}}{h} = \frac{8 \text{ mU}}{1 \text{ min}} \times \frac{1 \text{ U}}{1000 \text{ mU}} \times \frac{1000 \text{ cc}}{10 \text{ U}} \times \frac{60 \text{ min}}{1 \text{ h}}$$

Step 4: Cancel the labels that appear in both the numerator and the denominator on the same side of the equal sign.

$$\frac{x \text{ cc}}{h} = \frac{8}{1} \times \frac{1}{1000} \times \frac{1000 \text{ cc}}{10} \times \frac{60}{1 \text{ h}}$$

Step 5: Complete the required mathematical operations.

$$\frac{x \text{ cc}}{h} = \frac{48 \text{ cc}}{h}$$

Therefore, the rate is 48 cc/h.

▶ SOLVED PRACTICE PROBLEMS

1. The order is for 12 milliunits of Pitocin (oxytocin) per minute. The IV of 500 cc contains 5 units of Pitocin. Determine the rate of the IV in gtts/min and cc/h using a drop factor of 10 gtts/cc.

$$\frac{x \text{ gtts}}{min} = \frac{12 \text{ mU}}{1 \text{ min}} \times \frac{1 \text{ U}}{1000 \text{ mU}} \times \frac{500 \text{ cc}}{5 \text{ U}} \times \frac{10 \text{ gtts}}{1 \text{ cc}}$$

$$\frac{x \text{ cc}}{h} = \frac{12 \text{ mU}}{1 \text{ min}} \times \frac{1 \text{ U}}{1000 \text{ mU}} \times \frac{500 \text{ cc}}{5 \text{ U}} \times \frac{60 \text{ min}}{1 \text{ h}}$$

▶ **Answer:** 12 gtts/min and 72 cc/h

2. The patient is to receive IV heparin at a rate of 1000 units per hour. The IV has been prepared with 24,000 units of heparin per liter. Using a drop factor of 60 gtts/cc, determine the rate in gtts/min and cc/h.

$$\frac{x \text{ gtts}}{min} = \frac{1000 \text{ U}}{1 \text{ h}} \times \frac{1000 \text{ cc}}{24,000 \text{ U}} \times \frac{60 \text{ gtts}}{1 \text{ cc}} \times \frac{1 \text{ h}}{60 \text{ min}}$$

$$\frac{x \text{ cc}}{h} = \frac{1000 \text{ U}}{1 \text{ h}} \times \frac{1000 \text{ cc}}{24,000 \text{ U}}$$

▶ **Answer:** 42 gtts/min and 42 cc/h.

3. The patient is to receive morphine sulfate IV 9 mg per hour. The IV is 200 mg of morphine in 1000 cc of fluid. Using 60 gtts/cc, calculate the rate in gtts/min.

$$\frac{x \text{ gtts}}{min} = \frac{9 \text{ mg}}{1 \text{ h}} \times \frac{1000 \text{ cc}}{200 \text{ mg}} \times \frac{60 \text{ gtts}}{1 \text{ cc}} \times \frac{1 \text{ h}}{60 \text{ min}}$$

▶ **Answer:** 45 gtts/min

4. The order is to give lidocaine 2 mg/min using an IV of 1 g of lidocaine per 500 cc of 5% dextrose. Using a drop factor of 60 gtts/cc, determine the rate in gtts/min and cc/h.

$$\frac{x \text{ gtts}}{\min} = \frac{2 \text{ mg}}{1 \min} \times \frac{1 \text{ g}}{1000 \text{ mg}} \times \frac{500 \text{ cc}}{1 \text{ g}} \times \frac{60 \text{ gtts}}{1 \text{ cc}}$$

$$\frac{x \text{ cc}}{h} = \frac{2 \text{ mg}}{1 \min} \times \frac{1 \text{ g}}{1000 \text{ mg}} \times \frac{500 \text{ cc}}{1 \text{ g}} \times \frac{60 \min}{1 \text{ h}}$$

▶ **Answer:** 60 gtts/min and 60 cc/h

5. The patient is to receive Isuprel (isoproterenol) at a rate of 4 μg/min. The concentration of the Isuprel is 2 mg per 500 cc of IV fluid. Using a drop factor of 60 gtts/cc, find the rate in gtts/min and cc/h.

$$\frac{x \text{ gtts}}{\min} = \frac{4 \text{ } \mu g}{\min} \times \frac{1 \text{ mg}}{1000 \text{ } \mu g} \times \frac{500 \text{ cc}}{2 \text{ mg}} \times \frac{60 \text{ gtts}}{1 \text{ cc}}$$

$$\frac{x \text{ cc}}{h} = \frac{4 \text{ mcg}}{\min} \times \frac{1 \text{ mg}}{1000 \text{ } \mu g} \times \frac{500 \text{ cc}}{2 \text{ mg}} \times \frac{60 \min}{1 \text{ h}}$$

▶ **Answer:** 60 gtts/min and 60 cc/h

Calculation of Dosage

It is not uncommon for physicians to order the rate of a continuous IV medication in cubic centimeters per hour without indicating the exact dosage of the drug that the patient is receiving. Since it is the nurse's responsibility to know the dosage being administered, the nurse should know how to calculate the amount of medication the patient is receiving per minute or per hour.

Example 9.6: The order is to give heparin 25,000 units in 1000 cc of IV fluid at a rate of 40 cc/h. Determine how many U/h the patient is receiving.

Step 1: State the problem in equation form.

$$\frac{x \text{ U}}{h} = \frac{40 \text{ cc}}{h}$$

Step 2: Identify the conversion factor needed to convert from cubic centimeters per hour to units per hour. The information needed from the problem to identify the conversion factor is: There are 25,000 units per 1000 cc of IV fluid (25,000 U = 1000 cc).

Step 3: Put into the equation the form of the conversion factor that will cancel the unwanted labels and leave only the desired labels on both sides of the equal sign.

$$\frac{x \text{ U}}{h} = \frac{40 \text{ cc}}{h} \times \frac{25,000 \text{ U}}{1000 \text{ cc}}$$

Step 4: Cancel the labels that appear in both the numerator and the denominator on the same side of the equal sign.

$$\frac{x \text{ U}}{h} = \frac{40}{h} \times \frac{25,000 \text{ U}}{1000}$$

Step 5: Complete the required mathematical operations.

$$\frac{x \text{ U}}{h} = \frac{1000 \text{ U}}{h}$$

Therefore, the patient is receiving 1000 U/h.

Example 9.7: The patient is to receive aminophylline at a rate of 20 cc/h. The concentration of medication is 500 mg per 1000 cc of IV fluid. Determine how many mg/h the patient is receiving.

Step 1: State the problem in equation form.

$$\frac{x\,mg}{h} = \frac{20\,cc}{h}$$

Step 2: Identify the conversion factor needed to convert from cubic centimeter per hour to milligrams per hour. The information needed from the problem to identify the conversion factor is: There are 500 mg per 1000 cc of IV fluid (500 mg = 1000 cc).

Step 3: Put into the equation the form of the conversion factor that will cancel the unwanted labels and leave only the desired labels on both sides of the equal sign.

$$\frac{x\,mg}{h} = \frac{20\,cc}{h} \times \frac{500\,mg}{1000\,cc}$$

Step 4: Cancel the labels that appear in both the numerator and the denominator on the same side of the equal sign.

$$\frac{x\,mg}{h} = \frac{20}{h} \times \frac{500\,mg}{1000}$$

Step 5: Complete the required mathematical operations.

$$\frac{x\,mg}{h} = \frac{10\,mg}{h}$$

Therefore, the patient is receiving 10 mg/h.

Example 9.8: The patient is receiving lidocaine at 40 cc/h. The concentration of the medication is 1 gram per 500 cc of IV fluid. Determine how many mg/min the patient is receiving.

Step 1: State the problem in equation form.

$$\frac{x\,mg}{min} = \frac{40\,cc}{h}$$

Step 2: Identify the conversion factors needed to convert from cubic centimeters per hour to milligrams per minute. The information needed from the problem to identify the conversion factors is: There is 1 gram per 500 cc of IV fluid.

Three conversion factors are used:

A. Convert from cubic centimeters to grams.

500 cc = 1 g

B. Convert from grams to milligrams.

1 g = 1000 mg

C. Convert from hours to minutes.

1 h = 60 min

Step 3: Put into the equation the form of each conversion factor that will cancel the unwanted labels and leave only the desired labels on both sides of the equal sign.

$$\frac{x \, mg}{min} = \frac{40 \, cc}{h} \times \frac{1 \, g}{500 \, cc} \times \frac{1000 \, mg}{1 \, g} \times \frac{1 \, h}{60 \, min}$$

Step 4: Cancel the labels that appear in both the numerator and the denominator on the same side of the equal sign.

$$\frac{x \, mg}{min} = \frac{40}{1} \times \frac{1}{500} \times \frac{1000 \, mg}{1} \times \frac{1}{60 \, min}$$

Step 5: Complete the required mathematical operations.

$$\frac{x \, mg}{min} = \frac{1.33 \, mg}{min}$$

Therefore, the patient is receiving 1.33 mg/min.

► SOLVED PRACTICE PROBLEMS

1. The order is Pitocin (oxytocin) 5 units per 500 cc of IV fluid at 66 cc/h. Determine how many mU/min the patient is receiving.

$$\frac{x \, mU}{min} = \frac{66 \, cc}{h} \times \frac{5 \, U}{500 \, cc} \times \frac{1000 \, mU}{1 \, U} \times \frac{1 \, h}{60 \, min}$$

► **Answer:** 11 mU/min

2. The patient is receiving heparin 50 ml/h with a concentration of 26,000 units per liter. Determine how many U/h the patient is receiving.

$$\frac{x \, U}{h} = \frac{50 \, ml}{h} \times \frac{26,000 \, U}{1 \, L} \times \frac{1 \, L}{1000 \, ml}$$

► **Answer:** 1300 U/h

3. The order is Isuprel (isoproterenol) at a rate of 30 cc/h. The concentration of the IV is 1 mg per 250 cc of IV fluid. Determine how many μg/min the patient is receiving.

$$\frac{x \, \mu g}{min} = \frac{30 \, cc}{h} \times \frac{1 \, mg}{250 \, cc} \times \frac{1000 \, \mu g}{1 \, mg} \times \frac{1 \, h}{60 \, min}$$

► **Answer:** 2 μg/min

4. The order is morphine sulfate 80 mg in 250 cc of IV fluid to infuse at a rate of 20 cc/h. Determine how many mg/h the patient is receiving.

$$\frac{x \, mg}{h} = \frac{20 \, cc}{h} \times \frac{80 \, mg}{250 \, cc}$$

► **Answer:** 6.4 mg/h

5. The patient is receiving Pitocin (oxytocin) 10 units per 1000 cc at a rate of 40 cc/h. Determine how many mU/min the patient is receiving.

$$\frac{x\,\text{mU}}{\text{min}} = \frac{40\,\text{cc}}{\text{h}} \times \frac{10\,\text{U}}{1000\,\text{cc}} \times \frac{1000\,\text{mU}}{1\,\text{U}} \times \frac{1\,\text{h}}{60\,\text{min}}$$

▶ **Answer:** 6.67 mU/min

CASE STUDY

▶ Case Nine

K.M., a 54-year-old male, was admitted with a diagnosis of pneumonia. He has a history of chronic obstructive pulmonary disease (COPD). Among his current medical orders are: elevate head of bed 45 degrees; oxygen at 2 L/min per nasal canula; IV aminophylline 750 mg in 1000 cc D$_5$W at 50 mg/h; ticarcillin 1 g IVPB via heparin lock q6h.

The ordered medications are labeled as follows:

Pharmacy Computer Printout Label

Name: K.M.	**Room 226**	**Date:** 09/16/xx
Order:	ticarcillin 1 Gm IVPB	
Supplied:	1 gram per 50 cc D$_5$W	
Directions:	Administer over 30 min–2 hours	

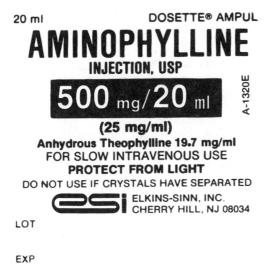

Refer to the medication labels to answer the following questions.

1. How many cc of aminophylline must be added to 1000 cc of D$_5$W to produce the ordered concentration?
2. What rate (cc/h) is needed to administer 50 mg of aminophylline per hour?
3. Using minidrop tubing, how many gtts/min are needed to administer the aminophylline?

4. The ticarcillin piggyback contains how many cc of IV fluid?
5. What is the minimum infusion time for the ticarcillin?
6. What is the maximum infusion time for the ticarcillin?
7. Using an infusion set that delivers 15 gtts/cc, determine the gtts/min needed to administer the ticarcillin over:
   A. 30 minutes
   B. 1 hour
   C. 2 hours

For answers to Case Study Nine, see page 171.

► SELF-TEST

1. The order is to give Mandol (cefamandole) 1 g q6h IVPB. Recommended dilution is 50–100 cc of compatible IV fluid. Recommended rate of administration is 15–30 minutes. Using 10 gtts/cc, determine the gtts/min needed to give a 100 cc piggyback in 30 minutes.
2. The order is to give Aldomet (methyldopa) 250 mg q6h IVPB. The medication is diluted in 100 cc of 5% dextrose. Using 60 gtts/cc, find the rate in gtts/min needed to give the Aldomet over 1 hour.
3. The physician has ordered garamycin 80 mg q8h IVPB. The medication is dissolved in 150 ml of normal saline. Using 20 gtts/cc, find the rate in gtts/min needed to give the medication in 45 minutes.
4. The order is for oxacillin 500 mg q6h IVPB. The medication is dissolved in 50 cc of IV fluid. Using a drop factor of 10 gtts/cc, find the rate in gtts/min needed to give the drug in 15 minutes.
5. The patient is to receive 100 mg of Vibramycin q12h IVPB dissolved in 500 cc of IV fluid. The medication is to be infused over 3 hours. Determine the rate of the IV in cc/h.
6. The patient is to receive 250 ml of Albuminar-5 (normal serum albumin) at the rate of 0.25 grams per minute. The concentration of the Albuminar-5 is 5 g per 100 ml. Using a drop factor of 10 gtts/cc, determine the rate in gtts/min.
7. The order is to infuse Isuprel (isoproterenol) at a rate of 3 μg per minute. The concentration of Isuprel is 2 mg per 250 cc IV fluid. Using 60 gtts/cc, find the rate of infusion in gtts/min and cc/h.
8. The order is to infuse Levophed (levarterenol) at a rate of 4 μg per minute. The concentration of the IV is 8 mg of Levophed per 250 cc. Find the rate of infusion in cc/h.
9. The patient is to receive heparin at a rate of 1500 units per hour. The IV has 30,000 U per 500 cc of 5% dextrose. Find the rate in cc/h.
10. The order is to give IV heparin 1100 units per hour. The IV contains 26,000 units of heparin per liter. Determine the rate of the IV in cc/h.
11. The patient is to receive Pitocin (oxytocin) at a rate of 16 milliunits per minute. The IV contains 10 units of Pitocin in 1000 cc. Using a drop factor of 60 gtts/cc, find the rate in gtts/min and cc/h.

Continued next page

▶ **Self-Test Continued**

12. The patient is to receive 10 milliunits of Pitocin (oxytocin) per minute. The IV contains 10 units of Pitocin in 1 liter of 5% dextrose. Determine the rate of the IV in gtts/min and cc/h using a drop factor of 60 gtts/cc.
13. The patient is receiving aminophylline at 40 cc/h. The concentration of the medication is 500 mg per 1000 cc. Determine how many mg/h the patient is receiving.
14. The order is to add 100 mg of morphine to 500 cc of IV fluid and administer at a rate of 30 cc/h. Determine how many mg/h the patient is receiving.
15. The order is to administer lidocaine at a rate of 30 cc/h using a concentration of 4 mg/cc. Determine how many mg/min the patient is receiving.

For answers to the self-test, see below.

ANSWERS
to Case Study Nine

ANSWERS
to Self-test

1. 30 cc
2. 67 cc/h
3. 67 gtts/min

4. 50 cc
5. 30 min
6. 2 h

7. A. 25 gtts/min
   B. 13 gtts/min
   C. 6 gtts/min

1. 33 gtts/min
2. 100 gtts/min
3. 67 gtts/min
4. 33 gtts/min
5. 167 cc/h

6. 50 gtts/min
7. 23 gtts/min and 23 cc/h
8. 8 cc/h
9. 25 cc/h
10. 42 cc/h

11. 96 gtts/min and 96 cc/h
12. 60 gtts/min and 60 cc/h
13. 20 mg/h
14. 6 mg/h
15. 2 mg/min

Pediatric Intravenous Medications

▲ OBJECTIVES

Upon completion of Chapter 10, the student will be able to:

▷ Calculate the volume of IV medication solution needed to supply the amount of medication ordered.

▷ Determine how much total solution is needed with the ordered dose to produce the recommended pediatric concentration.

▷ Calculate the rate of infusion needed to administer the medication in the amount of time recommended for infusion.

▲ INTRODUCTION TO PEDIATRIC INTRAVENOUS ANTIBIOTICS

Dilution of medications for IV administration to pediatric patients must follow strict guidelines to produce concentrations that are not irritating to veins. Moreover, the volume of fluid used in IV administration to pediatric patients is restricted; therefore, the minimum allowable dilution must be determined. Pediatric nursing units usually have guidelines for preparation of antibiotic solutions. In the examples given in this chapter, generally accepted guidelines are used.

This chapter describes the steps to follow to produce a solution with the recommended concentration for administration to pediatric patients. It should be noted that the recommended concentration is the maximum allowed concentration and it requires the minimum allowed dilution in its preparation. Depending on the size and condition of the patient, the medication may be further diluted to provide a larger volume of solution to infuse. Increasing the dilution will decrease the concentration of the medication in the solution.

As in previous chapters, calculations needed to prepare the appropriate concentration for pediatric IV medications are carried out using the dimensional analysis method of problem solving discussed in Chapter 2. As noted below (Part 1, steps 1 and 2) a two-part calculation is used to determine how to prepare the maximum allowed concentration. Following the determination of the maximum allowed concentration, the IV rate is calculated (Part 2) using the method discussed in Chapter 8 (refer to Chapter 8 for review if necessary).

► alert:

It is *permissible* to administer a solution of *lower* concentration than recommended provided the patient can tolerate the added fluid; however, it is *not permissible* to administer solutions of *higher* concentration than recommended.

► critical decision point:

The order reads: *Vancomycin 250 mg IVPB q6h.* The patient is a 60 lb child. The medication concentration guidelines used in your pediatric unit indicate a maximum recommended concentration of 5 mg/ml for vancomycin. A nurse who is being oriented to your unit tells you that she has reconstituted a 1 gram vial of vancomycin by adding 20 ml of sterile water for injection. She also tells you that the resulting solution has a concentration of 50 mg/ml. The nurses asks you if the ordered dose of 250 mg of vancomycin can be diluted to 100 ml in a buretrol with compatible IV fluid.

► decision/action:

Since the concentration of vancomycin is 50 mg/ml, you determine that 5 ml is needed to provide the ordered dose of 250 mg. You realize that diluting 250 mg of vancomycin with enough IV fluid to produce 50 ml of solution will yield the maximum recommended concentration of 5 mg/ml (250 mg/50 ml = 5 mg/ml). Therefore, you recognize that adding a *larger* amount of IV fluid will create a *lower* concentration. You tell the nurse that adding enough IV fluid to 250 mg of vancomycin to produce 100 ml of solution would yield a concentration of 2.5 mg/ml (250 mg/100 ml = 2.5 mg/ml). Since this concentration is *less than* the maximum recommended concentration for pediatric patients, you advise the nurse that it may be used for this patient.

Finding the Maximum Allowed Concentration and Recommended Rate of Infusion

Part 1: Maximum Allowed Concentration

1. Calculate the volume (ml) of the medication solution needed to supply the amount (e.g., mg or units) of the medication ordered.
2. Determine how much *total solution* (ml) is needed with the ordered dose (e.g., mg or units) to produce the recommended pediatric concentration.

Part 2: Recommended Infusion Rate
Calculate the rate of infusion needed to administer the medication solution in the time required.

▲ MEDICATIONS AVAILABLE IN SOLUTION FORM

Example 10.1: The physician ordered Garamycin (gentamicin) 25 mg IVPB q8h for a 13.5 kg infant.

The medication is supplied in solution form in 20 mg vials with a concentration of 10 mg/ml.

The guidelines of the pediatric nursing unit for administration of Garamycin are: recommended concentration 2 mg/ml and duration of infusion 15–30 minutes.

Information Summary

Medication: Garamycin

Amount ordered: 25 mg

How supplied: 20 mg vials

Available concentration: 10 mg/ml

Recommended infusion time:
  15–30 minutes

Recommended concentration:
  2 mg/ml

Part 1: Maximum Allowed Concentration

1. Calculate the volume (ml) of medication solution needed to supply the amount (mg) of medication ordered.

   The question asked is: How many ml of solution equal 25 mg of Garamycin if 1 ml contains 10 mg? (Conversion factor: 1 ml = 10 mg.)

   Stated in equation form:

   $$x \text{ ml} = 25 \text{ mg} \times \frac{1 \text{ ml}}{10 \text{ mg}}$$

   $$x \text{ ml} = 2.5 \text{ ml}$$

   Therefore, 2.5 ml of solution contains 25 mg of Garamycin.

2. Determine how much total solution (ml) is needed for the ordered dose (i.e., 25 mg) to produce the recommended concentration.

   Recall that the recommended concentration is 2 mg/ml and the amount of medication to administer is 25 mg.

   The question asked is: How many ml are needed with 25 mg of Garamycin if 1 ml is needed per 2 mg? (Conversion factor: 1 ml = 2 mg.)

   Stated in equation form:

   $$x \text{ ml} = 25 \text{ mg} \times \frac{1 \text{ ml}}{2 \text{ mg}}$$

   $$x \text{ ml} = 12.5 \text{ ml}$$

   Therefore, 12.5 ml is the total amount of solution needed for dilution of 25 mg of Garamycin.

Summary

To prepare the maximum accepted concentration with the minimum amount of dilution, add to 2.5 ml of Garamycin solution enough compatible diluent to give a total final volume of 12.5 ml of solution. The 12.5 ml of solution will contain 25 mg of Garamycin and have a concentration of 2 mg/ml.

The actual procedure to follow in the preparation of the Garamycin solution using a volume control set such as a buretrol is illustrated in Figure 10–1.

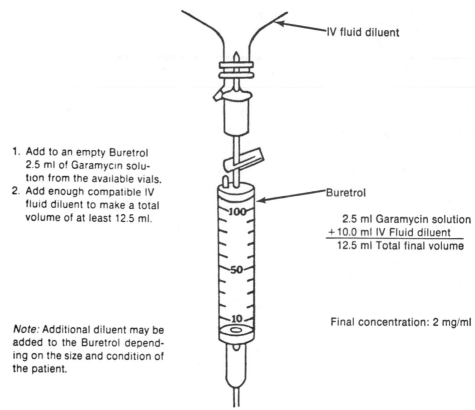

1. Add to an empty Buretrol 2.5 ml of Garamycin solution from the available vials.
2. Add enough compatible IV fluid diluent to make a total volume of at least 12.5 ml.

IV fluid diluent

Buretrol

2.5 ml Garamycin solution
+10.0 ml IV Fluid diluent
12.5 ml Total final volume

Note: Additional diluent may be added to the Buretrol depending on the size and condition of the patient.

Final concentration: 2 mg/ml

FIGURE 10–1. Dilution of Garamycin in a Buretrol.

Part 2: Recommended Infusion Rate
Calculate the rate of infusion needed to administer the solution of medication in the time required.

Note: As a general rule, pediatric IV infusions are administered with IV tubing having a drop factor of 60 gtts/ml.

Recall that the recommended time of infusion for Garamycin is 15–30 minutes. To illustrate the calculation necessary, the maximum time of infusion will be used. The total amount of solution to be infused is 12.5 ml.

The question asked is: How many drops per minute are required to administer 12.5 ml of solution in 30 minutes using an infusion set with a drop factor of 60 gtts/ml? (Conversion factor: 60 gtts = 1 ml.)

Stated in equation form:

$$\frac{x \text{ gtts}}{\text{min}} = \frac{12.5 \text{ ml}}{30 \text{ min}} \times \frac{60 \text{ gtts}}{1 \text{ ml}}$$

$$\frac{x \text{ gtts}}{\text{min}} = \frac{25 \text{ gtts}}{1 \text{ min}}$$

Therefore, 25 gtts/min will infuse 12.5 ml of Garamycin solution in 30 minutes.

▲ MEDICATIONS REQUIRING RECONSTITUTION

Example 10.2: The physician ordered ampicillin 350 mg IVPB q4h for a 10.8 kg infant.

The medication is supplied as a dry powder in 500-mg vials. Directions for reconstitution of the medication state: "Add 1.8 ml of diluent to produce a withdrawable volume of 2 ml with a concentration of 250 mg/ml."

The guidelines of the pediatric nursing unit for administration of ampicillin are: recommended concentration for an infant 50 mg/ml and for a child 100 mg/ml; duration of infusion 10–20 minutes.

First, reconstitute the medication as directed by adding 1.8 ml of compatible diluent. The resulting concentration is 250 mg/ml. Recall that with reconstituted medications, the final concentration is used in calculations of dosage.

Data Summary

Medication: Ampicillin	Amount ordered: 350 mg
How supplied: 500-mg vials	Available concentration: 250 mg/ml
Recommended infusion time: 10–20 minutes	Recommended concentration: 50 mg/ml

Part 1: Maximum Allowed Concentration

1. Calculate the volume (ml) of medication solution needed to supply the amount (mg) of medication ordered.

   The question asked is: How many ml of solution equal 350 mg of ampicillin if 1 ml contains 250 mg? (Conversion factor: 1 ml = 250 mg.)

   Stated in equation form:

   $$x \text{ ml} = 350 \text{ mg} \times \frac{1 \text{ ml}}{250 \text{ mg}}$$

   $$x \text{ ml} = 1.4 \text{ ml}$$

   Therefore, 1.4 ml of solution contains 350 mg of ampicillin.

2. Determine how much total solution (ml) is needed for the ordered dose (i.e., 350 mg) to produce the recommended concentration.

   The question asked is: How many ml are needed with 350 mg of ampicillin if 1 ml is needed per 50 mg? (Conversion factor: 1ml = 50 mg.)

   Stated in equation form:

   $$x \text{ ml} = 350 \text{ mg} \times \frac{1 \text{ ml}}{50 \text{ mg}}$$

   $$x \text{ ml} = 7 \text{ ml}$$

   Therefore, 7 ml is the total amount of solution needed for dilution of 350 mg of ampicillin.

Summary

To prepare the maximum accepted concentration with the minimum amount of dilution, add to 1.4 ml of ampicillin solution enough compatible diluent to give a total final volume of 7 ml of solution. The 7 ml of solution will contain 350 mg of ampicillin and have a concentration of 50 mg/ml.

Note: This solution may be further diluted depending on the size and clinical condition of the patient.

Part 2: Recommended Infusion Rate
Calculate the rate of infusion needed to administer the solution of medication in the time required.

The recommended time of infusion for ampicillin is 10–20 minutes; in this calculation the maximum time will be used.

The question asked is: How many drops per minute are required to administer 7 ml of solution in 20 minutes using an infusion set with a drop factor of 60 gtts/ml? (Conversion factor: 60 gtts = 1 ml.)

Stated in equation form:

$$\frac{x \text{ gtts}}{\text{min}} = \frac{7 \text{ ml}}{20 \text{ min}} \times \frac{60 \text{ gtts}}{1 \text{ ml}}$$

$$\frac{x \text{ gtts}}{\text{min}} = \frac{21 \text{ gtts}}{1 \text{ min}}$$

Therefore, 21 gtts/min will infuse 7 ml of ampicillin solution in 20 minutes.

Example 10.3: The order is penicillin G 300,000 units IVPB q4h for a 7.5 kg infant.

The medication is available in powder form in 5 million–unit vials. Directions for reconstitution of the medication are:

PENICILLIN G CONCENTRATION	VOLUME OF DILUENT TO BE ADDED	WITHDRAWABLE VOLUME
200,000 units/ml	23 ml	25 ml
250,000 units/ml	18 ml	20 ml
500,000 units/ml	8 ml	10 ml
1,000,000 units/ml	3 ml	5 ml

The guidelines of the pediatric nursing unit for the administration of penicillin G are: recommended concentration for infants 50,000 units/ml and for large children 250,000 units/ml; duration of infusion 10–20 minutes.

First, determine which reconstitution directions could be used. If the desired concentration is not in the reconstitution table provided by the manufacturer, any *higher* concentration *may be used*. Concentrations *lower* than the desired are too diluted and *cannot be used*.

In this problem any of the concentrations listed may be used since all are *higher* than the recommended concentration. The problem is solved using 200,000 units/ml.

Data Summary

Medication: Penicillin G

How supplied: 5,000,000 unit vials

Recommended infusion time: 10–20 minutes

Amount ordered: 300,000 units

Available concentration: 200,000 units/ml

Recommended concentration: 50,000 units/ml

Part 1: Maximum Allowed Concentration

1. Calculate the volume (ml) of medication solution needed to supply the amount (mg) of medication ordered.

   The question asked is: How many ml of solution equal 300,000 units of penicillin G if 1 ml contains 200,000 units? (Conversion factor: 1 ml = 200,000 U.)

   Stated in equation form:

   $$x\,ml = 300{,}000\;U \times \frac{1\;ml}{200{,}000\;U}$$

   $$x\,ml = 1.5\;ml$$

   Therefore, 1.5 ml of solution contains 300,000 U of penicillin G.

2. Determine how much total solution (ml) is needed for the ordered dose (i.e., 300,000 units) to produce the recommended concentration.

   The question asked is: How many ml are needed with 300,000 units of penicillin G if 1 ml is needed per 50,000 units? (Conversion factor: 1 ml = 50,000 U.)

   Stated in equation form:

   $$x\,ml = 300{,}000\;U \times \frac{1\;ml}{50{,}000\;U}$$

   $$x\,ml = 6\;ml$$

   Therefore, 6 ml is the total amount of solution needed for dilution of 300,000 U of penicillin G.

Summary

To prepare the maximum accepted concentration with the minimum amount of dilution, add to 1.5 ml of penicillin G solution enough compatible diluent to give a total final volume of 6 ml of solution. The 6 ml of solution will contain 300,000 U of penicillin G and have a concentration of 50,000 U/ml.

Note: This solution may be further diluted depending on the size and the clinical condition of the patient.

Part 2: Recommended Infusion Rate

Calculate the rate of infusion needed to administer the solution of medication in the time required.

The question asked is: How many drops per minute are required to administer 6 ml of solution in 20 minutes using an infusion set with a drop factor of 60 gtts/ml? (Conversion factor: 60 gtts = 1 ml.)

Stated in equation form:

$$\frac{x \text{ gtts}}{\text{min}} = \frac{6 \text{ ml}}{20 \text{ min}} \times \frac{60 \text{ gtts}}{1 \text{ ml}}$$

$$\frac{x \text{ gtts}}{\text{min}} = \frac{18 \text{ gtts}}{1 \text{ min}}$$

Therefore, 18 gtts/min will infuse 6 ml of penicillin G solution in 20 minutes.

▶ SOLVED PRACTICE PROBLEMS

1. The physician ordered Unipen (nafcillin) 900 mg IVPB q6h for a 27 kg child. The medication is supplied as a dry powder in 1 gram vials. Directions for reconstitution of the medication state: "Add 3.4 ml of diluent to produce a 1 g/4 ml solution with a concentration of 250 mg/ml." The guidelines for administration of nafcillin are: concentration 100 mg/ml and duration of infusion 10–20 minutes.

    A. How many ml of solution contain 900 mg of nafcillin if 4 ml = 1 g?

    $$x \text{ ml} = 900 \text{ mg} \times \frac{4 \text{ ml}}{1 \text{ g}} \times \frac{1 \text{ g}}{1000 \text{ mg}}$$

    Therefore, 3.6 ml of solution contains 900 mg of nafcillin.

    ▶ **Answer:** $x \text{ ml} = 3.6 \text{ ml}$

    B. How much total solution is needed for 900 mg of nafcillin to produce a concentration of 100 mg/ml?

    $$x \text{ ml} = 900 \text{ mg} \times \frac{1 \text{ ml}}{100 \text{ mg}}$$

    Therefore, to 3.6 ml of nafcillin solution (900 mg) add enough diluent to give a total final volume of 9 ml.

    ▶ **Answer:** $x \text{ ml} = 9 \text{ ml}$

    C. At what rate should the IV be run to complete the 9 ml medication infusion in 20 minutes?

    $$\frac{x \text{ gtts}}{\text{min}} = \frac{9 \text{ ml}}{20 \text{ min}} \times \frac{60 \text{ gtts}}{1 \text{ ml}}$$

    Therefore, 27 gtts/min will infuse the solution in 20 minutes.

    ▶ **Answer:** $\dfrac{x \text{ gtts}}{\text{min}} = \dfrac{27 \text{ gtts}}{1 \text{ min}}$

2. The order is Prostaphlin (oxacillin) 325 mg IVPB q6h for a 13-kg infant. The medication is supplied in 500-mg vials. Directions for reconstitution of the medication state: "Add 2.8 ml of diluent to the vial to produce a final volume of 3 ml." The guidelines for administration of oxacillin are: concentration 50 mg/ml and duration of infusion 30 minutes.

A. How many ml of solution contain 325 mg of oxacillin if 3 ml = 500 mg?

$$x \text{ ml} = 325 \text{ mg} \times \frac{3 \text{ ml}}{500 \text{ mg}}$$

Therefore, 1.95 ml of solution contains 325 mg of oxacillin.

▶ **Answer:** x ml = 1.95 ml

B. How much total solution is needed for 325 mg of oxacillin to produce a concentration of 50 mg/ml?

$$x \text{ ml} = 325 \text{ mg} \times \frac{1 \text{ ml}}{50 \text{ mg}}$$

Therefore, to 1.95 ml of oxacillin solution (325 mg) add enough diluent to give a total final volume of 6.5 ml.

▶ **Answer:** x ml = 6.5 ml

C. At what rate should the IV be run to complete the 6.5 ml medication infusion in 30 minutes?

$$\frac{x \text{ gtts}}{\text{min}} = \frac{6.5 \text{ ml}}{30 \text{ min}} \times \frac{60 \text{ gtts}}{1 \text{ ml}}$$

Therefore, 13 gtts/min will infuse the solution in 30 minutes.

▶ **Answer:** $\dfrac{x \text{ gtts}}{\text{min}} = \dfrac{13 \text{ gtts}}{1 \text{ min}}$

3. The order is to give Cleocin (clindamycin) 120 mg IVPB q8h to a 19 kg child. The medication is supplied in vials with 300 mg per 2 ml. The guidelines for administration of clindamycin are: concentration 6 mg/ml and duration of infusion 15–30 minutes.

A. How many ml of solution contain 120 mg of clindamycin if 2 ml = 300 mg?

$$x \text{ ml} = 120 \text{ mg} \times \frac{2 \text{ ml}}{300 \text{ mg}}$$

Therefore, 0.8 ml of solution contains 120 mg of clindamycin.

▶ **Answer:** x ml = 0.8 ml

B. How much total solution is needed for 120 mg of clindamycin to produce a concentration of 6 mg/ml?

$$x \text{ ml} = 120 \text{ mg} \times \frac{1 \text{ ml}}{6 \text{ mg}}$$

Therefore, to 0.8 ml of clindamycin solution (120 mg) add enough diluent to give a total final volume of 20 ml.

▶ **Answer:** x ml = 20 ml

C. At what rate should the IV be run to complete the 20 ml antibiotic infusion in 30 minutes?

$$\frac{x \text{ gtts}}{\text{min}} = \frac{20 \text{ ml}}{30 \text{ min}} \times \frac{60 \text{ gtts}}{1 \text{ ml}}$$

Therefore, 40 gtts/min will infuse the solution in 30 minutes.

► Answer: $\dfrac{x \text{ gtts}}{\text{min}} = \dfrac{40 \text{ gtts}}{1 \text{ min}}$

CASE STUDY

► Case Ten

K.W. is a 19-month-old child admitted with a 3-day history of upper respiratory tract infection. K.W. weighs 24.5 lb. Currently K.W. is febrile, irritable, and anorexic. She has grunting respirations and sternal retractions. Her current medical diagnosis is staphlococcal pneumonia. Among her medical orders are: nasotracheal suctioning prn; 40% oxygen per mist tent; Tylenol elixir 2 cc for temp 101F or greater; vital signs q4h; IV of 5% dextrose and Ringer's lactate at 30 cc/h; Prostaphlin 110 mg IV per buretrol q6h; I&O (weigh all diapers).

The guidelines of the pediatric nursing unit for administration of Prostaphlin contain the following information.

IM INJECTION

VIAL SIZE	DILUENT	RESULTING CONCENTRATION
250 mg	1.4 cc	
500 mg	2.7 cc	250 mg/1.5 cc
1 g	5.7 cc	250 mg/1.5 cc
		250 mg/1.5 cc

IVPB (BURETROL)

Reconstitute the same as intramuscular.

Maximum recommended final concentration:

Infant: 50 mg/cc

Large child: 100 mg/cc

Infuse over 10–20 minutes.

Reconstitute with sterile water or sodium chloride injection.

Prostaphlin is sent from the pharmacy in a vial with the following label:

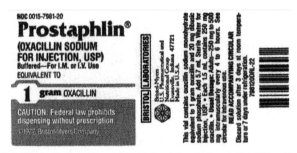

FIGURE 10–2. (Used with permission of Bristol Laboratories Division of Bristol-Myers Squibb Company, Syracuse, New York 13221-4755.)

Refer to the medication label and the guidelines for administration of Prostaphlin as needed to answer the following questions.

1. How many kilograms does the child weigh?
2. What diluent(s) can be used?
3. To reconstitute the powder, how much diluent should be added to the vial?
4. What is the concentration of the reconstituted solution?
5. For IV administration of Prostaphlin, what is the recommended final concentration for this child?
6. How many cc of Prostaphlin solution are needed to supply the ordered dose of 100 mg?
7. How much total solution is needed with the ordered dose to produce the maximum recommended pediatric concentration?
8. Calculate the rate of infusion needed to administer the medication solution over
   A. 10 minutes
   B. 20 minutes

For answers to Case Study Ten, see page 184.

▶ SELF-TEST

For each of the following problems calculate:

A. The volume (ml) of medication solution needed to supply the amount (e.g., mg or units) of the medication ordered.
B. How much total solution (ml) is needed with the ordered dose (e.g., mg or units) to produce the recommended concentration.
C. The rate of infusion needed to administer the solution of medication in the time required.

1. The physician ordered Amikin (amikacin) 165 mg q8h for a 33 kg child. The medication is supplied in vials containing 100 mg in 2 ml of solution. The guidelines for administration of amikacin are: concentration 6 mg/ml and duration of infusion 30–60 minutes.
2. The physician ordered Ancef (cefazolin) 475 mg q4h IVPB for a 19.6 kg child. The medication is supplied in 500 mg vials with a concentration of 250 mg/ml. The guidelines for administration of cefazolin are: concentration 50 mg/ml and duration of infusion 15–20 minutes.
3. The physician ordered Chloromycetin (chloramphenicol) 140 mg q6h for an 11.2 kg infant. The medication is supplied in a 1 gram vial. Reconstitution directions are: Add 10 ml of diluent to produce a concentration of 100 mg/ml. The guidelines for administration of chloramphenicol are: concentration 50 mg/ml and duration of infusion 10–20 minutes.
4. The physician ordered Ticar (ticarcillin) 700 mg q4h for a 41 kg child. The medication is supplied in a 1 gram vial. Reconstitution directions are: dilute with 4 ml to give an approximate concentration of 204

Continued next page

► Self-Test Continued

mg/ml. The guidelines for administration of ticarcillin are: concentration 100 mg/ml and duration of infusion 10–20 minutes.

5. The physician ordered Mandol (cefamandol) 450 mg q6h for a 22 kg child. The medication is supplied in a 500 mg vial. Reconstitution directions are: Add 4.75 ml of diluent to give a concentration of 100 mg/ml. The guidelines for administration of cefamandol are: concentration 50 mg/ml and duration of infusion 15–20 minutes.

6. The physician ordered Keflin (cephalothin) 480 mg q6h for a 19 kg child. The medication is supplied in a 1 gram vial. Reconstitution directions are: Add 5 ml of diluent to give a concentration of 500 mg per 2.7 ml. The guidelines for administration of cephalothin are: concentration 50 mg/ml and duration of infusion 15–20 minutes.

7. The physician ordered Vancocin (vancomycin) 240 mg q6h for a 52.0 lb child. The medication is supplied in 500 mg vials. Reconstitution directions are: Add 10 ml of diluent to give a concentration of 50 mg/ml. The guidelines for administration of vancomycin are: concentration 5 mg/ml and duration of infusion of 60 minutes.

8. The physician ordered penicillin G sodium 150,000 units q4h for an 8.8 kg infant. Refer to Example 10.3 for reconstitution directions and guidelines for administration.

9. The physician ordered penicillin G potassium 775,000 U q4h for an 18.6 kg infant. The medication is supplied in 1 million–unit vials. The reconstitution directions are given below. The guidelines for administration of penicillin G potassium are: concentration 250,000 U/ml and duration of infusion 10–20 minutes.

DILUENT	CONCENTRATION	TOTAL VOLUME
9.6 ml	100,000 U/ml	10 ml
4.6 ml	200,000 U/ml	5 ml
1.6 ml	500,000 U/ml	2 ml

10. The physician ordered Garamycin (gentamicin) 37.0 mg q8h for a 15 kg child. The medication is supplied in 20 mg vials with 10 mg/ml. The guidelines for administration of gentamicin are: concentration 10 mg/ml and duration of infusion 15–30 minutes.

For answers to the self-test, see page 185.

ANSWERS to Case Study Ten

1. 11.14 kg
2. Sterile water or sodium chloride injection
3. 1.4 cc
4. 25 mg/1.5 cc
5. 50 mg/cc
6. 0.66 cc
7. 2.2 cc
8. A. 13 gtts/min
   B. 7 gtts/min

1. A. 3.3 ml
   B. 27.5 ml
   C. 28 gtts/min
2. A. 1.9 ml
   B. 9.5 ml
   C. 29 gtts/min
3. A. 1.4 ml
   B. 2.8 ml
   C. 8 gtts/min
4. A. 3.4 ml
   B. 7 ml
   C. 21 gtts/min

5. A. 4.5 ml
   B. 9 ml
   C. 27 gtts/min
6. A. 2.6 ml
   B. 9.6 ml
   C. 29 gtts/min
7. A. 4.8 ml
   B. 48 ml
   C. 48 gtts/min
8. A. 0.75 ml
   B. 3 ml
   C. 9 gtts/min

9. A. 1.6 ml
   B. 3.1 ml
   C. 9 gtts/min
10. A. 3.7 ml
    B. 3.7 ml
    C. 7 gtts/min

ANSWERS to Self-test

IV Medications Based on Body Weight

11

▲ OBJECTIVES

Upon completion of Chapter 11, the student will be able to:

▶ Correctly calculate the rate of infusion in drops per minute or milliliters per hour needed to deliver a desired dosage of medication expressed in micrograms per kilogram per minutes (μg/kg/min) given:

The patient's weight in pounds or in kilograms
The concentration of the medication in the IV solution

▶ Correctly calculate the dosage of a medication the patient is receiving in micrograms per kilogram per minute (μg/kg/min) given:

The patient's weight in pounds or kilograms
The concentration of the medication in the IV solution
The current infusion rate in drops per minute or in milliliters per hour

▲ INTRODUCTION TO IV MEDICATIONS BASED ON BODY WEIGHT

Certain drugs that are given intravenously are extremely potent, and their administration requires careful monitoring. In some cases the nurse must be aware of the exact dosage (amount per kilogram per minute) that the patient is receiving. In these cases medication dosages are calculated on the basis of the patient's body weight. Administration of IV medications based on body weight usually requires constant nursing supervision, and as a result, patients receiving medications in this manner are often cared for in the critical care settings.

Physiologic responses to doses of intravenous medications that are based on body weight vary greatly from patient to patient. Particular medications also have different physiologic effects in varying dose ranges. The nurse must, therefore, be prepared to respond quickly and appropriately when there is a change in the patient's condition while receiving medications in this manner.

The rate of infusion and the dosage of these medications are critical; therefore, use of a mechanical IV infusion pump is preferred. The nurse's responsibility when administering medications in this manner is twofold: to calculate the flow rate of the medication, and then to determine the dosage the patient is receiving.

▲ CALCULATIONS WITH IV MEDICATIONS BASED ON BODY WEIGHT

The calculations in Chapter 11 deal with medications that are administered on the basis of micrograms per kilogram per minute (μg/kg/min). For medications given in this manner, minidrop tubing (drop factor of 60 gtts/cc) is used to provide greater control over the rate of administration. In addition, infusion pumps that measure cubic centimeters per hour are generally used, but the nurse should be prepared to calculate rates and dosages using either cubic centimeters per hour or drops per minute.

As in previous chapters, calculations of IV medications based on body weight are carried out using the dimensional analysis method of problem solving discussed in Chapter 2. The application of the method to IV medications based on body weight is illustrated below.

Example 11.1: The order is to give a 65 kg patient Intropin (dopamine) 8 micrograms per kilogram per minute (8μg/kg/min). The concentration of the medication is 400 mg in 500 cc of normal saline. Using a drop factor of 60 gtts/cc, determine the rate in gtts/min.

▶ Rules of Problem Solving by Dimensional Analysis

RULE 1 ▶

 One side of an equation can be multiplied by an appropriate conversion factor without changing the value of the equation.

▶ Application of Rule 1

When calculating IV medication rates and dosages based on weight, the following are considered to be conversion factors:

1. The concentration of the medication in the IV solution:

   In the problem given, the concentration of the medication is 400 mg in 500 cc. Therefore, the conversion factor is: 400 mg = 500 cc. This conversion factor can be put into the problem in either of two possible forms:

   $$\frac{400 \text{ mg}}{500 \text{ cc}} \quad \text{or} \quad \frac{500 \text{ cc}}{400 \text{ mg}}$$

2. The given weight of the patient receiving the medication:

   In the problem given, the patient weighs 65 kg. Therefore, the conversion factor is: 65 kg = wt. This conversion factor can be put into the problem in either of two possible forms:

$$\frac{65 \text{ kg}}{\text{wt}} \quad \text{or} \quad \frac{\text{wt}}{65 \text{ kg}}$$

3. The drop factor of the infusion set being used:

In the problem given, the drop factor is 60 gtts/cc. Therefore, the conversion factor is: 1 cc = 60 gtts. This conversion factor can be put into the problem in either of two possible forms:

$$\frac{60 \text{ gtts}}{1 \text{ cc}} \quad \text{or} \quad \frac{1 \text{ cc}}{60 \text{ gtts}}$$

 The problem is correctly set up when all labels cancel from both the numerator and the denominator except the labels that are desired in the answer.

◀ RULE 2

▶ Application of Rule 2

1. In the problem given, the question asked is how many drops per minute to give to a patient of the given weight in order to equal 8 micrograms per kilogram per minute.

2. Stated in equation form, the problem is:

$$\frac{x \text{ gtts}}{\text{min} \times \text{wt}} = \frac{8 \text{ } \mu\text{g}}{\text{kg} \times \text{min}}$$

3. The conversion factors required are put into the equation as fractions. The form of each fraction used is that which will cancel the unwanted labels (micrograms and kilograms) and leave only the desired labels (drops per minute per given weight) on both sides of the equal sign.

The conversion factors given in the problem are: 400 mg = 500 cc; wt = 65 kg; 1 cc = 60 gtts. An additional conversion factor relating milligrams and micrograms is needed. That conversion factor is: 1 mg = 1000 μg.

$$\frac{x \text{ gtts}}{\text{min} \times \text{wt}} = \frac{8 \text{ } \mu\text{g}}{\text{kg} \times \text{min}} \times \frac{1 \text{ mg}}{1000 \text{ } \mu\text{g}} \times \frac{500 \text{ cc}}{400 \text{ mg}} \times \frac{60 \text{ gtts}}{1 \text{ cc}} \times \frac{65 \text{ kg}}{\text{wt}}$$

4. Cancel all labels that appear in both the numerator and denominator on the same side of the equal sign.

$$\frac{x \text{ gtts}}{\text{min} \times \text{wt}} = \frac{8}{\text{min}} \times \frac{1}{1000} \times \frac{500}{400} \times \frac{60 \text{ gtts}}{1} \times \frac{65}{\text{wt}}$$

5. Completing the required mathematical operations gives:

$$\frac{x \text{ gtts}}{\text{min} \times \text{wt}} = \frac{39 \text{ gtts}}{\text{min} \times \text{wt}}$$

Therefore, the rate of the IV is 39 gtts/min.

The method of problem solving by dimensional analysis illustrated above is used throughout this chapter. For simplicity the method is reduced to the same five-step procedure used in previous chapters.

▲ CALCULATION OF IV RATES USING MICROGRAMS PER KILOGRAM PER MINUTE

Example 11.2: The order is to infuse Dobutrex (dobutamine) 250 mg in 250 cc of 5% dextrose at 3.5 μg/kg/min. The patient weights 70 kg. Using a drop factor of 60 gtts/cc, determine the rate in gtts/min.

Step 1: State the problem in equation form.

$$\frac{x \text{ gtts}}{\text{min} \times \text{wt}} = \frac{3.5 \ \mu\text{g}}{\text{kg} \times \text{min}}$$

Step 2: Identify the conversion factors needed to convert from μg/kg/min to gtts/min/wt. The information needed from the problem to identify the conversion factors is: There are 250 mg per 250 cc of IV fluid; there are 60 drops per cc; the patient weighs 70 kg.

Four conversion factors are used:

A. Convert from micrograms to milligrams.

   1000 μg = 1 mg

B. Convert from milligrams to cubic centimeters.

   250 mg = 250 cc

C. Convert from cubic centimeters to drops.

   1 cc = 60 gtts

D. Convert from kilograms to weight.

   70 kg = wt

Step 3: Put into the equation the form of each conversion factor that will cancel the unwanted labels (micrograms and kilograms) and leave only the desired labels (drops per minute per given weight) on both sides of the equal sign.

$$\frac{x \text{ gtts}}{\text{min} \times \text{wt}} = \frac{3.5 \ \mu\text{g}}{\text{kg} \times \text{min}} \times \frac{1 \text{ mg}}{1000 \ \mu\text{g}} \times \frac{250 \text{ cc}}{250 \text{ mg}} \times \frac{60 \text{ gtts}}{1 \text{ cc}} \times \frac{70 \text{ kg}}{\text{wt}}$$

Step 4: Cancel the labels that appear in both the numerator and the denominator on the same side of the equal sign.

$$\frac{x \text{ gtts}}{\text{min} \times \text{wt}} = \frac{3.5}{\text{min}} \times \frac{1}{1000} \times \frac{250}{250} \times \frac{60 \text{ gtts}}{1} \times \frac{70}{\text{wt}}$$

Step 5: Complete the required mathematical operations.

$$\frac{x \text{ gtts}}{\text{min} \times \text{wt}} = \frac{14.7 \text{ gtts}}{\text{min} \times \text{wt}}$$

Therefore, the rate is 15 gtts/min.

Example 11.3: The order is to give Intropin (dopamine) 8 μg/kg/min to a 180 lb patient. The concentration of the Intropin is 200 mg in 500 cc of 5% dextrose.

The resulting dilution is equivalent to 400 μg of Intropin per cc. Using a drop factor of 60 gtts/cc, determine the rate in cc/h.

Step 1: State the problem in equation form.

$$\frac{x \text{ cc}}{h \times wt} = \frac{8 \ \mu g}{kg \times min}$$

Step 2: Identify the conversion factors needed to convert from μg/kg/min to cc/h/wt. The information needed from the problem to identify the conversion factors is: There are 400 μg per cc of IV fluid; the patient weighs 180 lb.

Four conversion factors are used:

A. Convert from micrograms to cubic centimeters.

$$400 \ \mu g = 1 \text{ cc}$$

B. Convert from minutes to hours.

$$60 \text{ min} = 1 \text{ h}$$

C. Convert from kilograms to pounds.

$$1 \text{ kg} = 2.2 \text{ lb}$$

D. Convert from pounds to weight.

$$180 \text{ lb} = wt$$

Step 3: Put into the equation the form of each conversion factor that will cancel the unwanted labels and leave only the desired labels on both sides of the equal sign.

$$\frac{x \text{ cc}}{h \times wt} = \frac{8 \ \mu g}{kg \times min} \times \frac{1 \text{ cc}}{400 \ \mu g} \times \frac{60 \text{ min}}{1 \text{ h}} \times \frac{1 \text{ kg}}{2.2 \text{ lb}} \times \frac{180 \text{ lb}}{wt}$$

Step 4: Cancel the labels that appear in both the numerator and the denominator on the same side of the equal sign.

$$\frac{x \text{ cc}}{h \times wt} = \frac{8}{1} \times \frac{1 \text{ cc}}{400} \times \frac{60}{1 \text{ h}} \times \frac{1}{2.2} \times \frac{180}{wt}$$

Step 5: Complete the required mathematical operations.

$$\frac{x \text{ cc}}{h \times wt} = \frac{98 \text{ cc}}{h \times wt}$$

Therefore, the rate is 98 cc/h.

▶ SOLVED PRACTICE PROBLEMS

1. The order is to infuse Dobutrex (dobutamine) 250 mg in 200 ml of 5% dextrose solution at a rate of 8 μg/kg/min. The patient weighs 70 kg. Using a drop factor of 60 gtts/cc, determine the rate in gtts/min.

$$\frac{x \text{ gtts}}{min \times wt} = \frac{8 \ \mu g}{kg \times min} \times \frac{1 \text{ mg}}{1000 \ \mu g} \times \frac{200 \text{ ml}}{250 \text{ mg}} \times \frac{60 \text{ gtts}}{1 \text{ ml}} \times \frac{70 \text{ kg}}{wt}$$

▶ **Answer:** 27 gtts/min

2. The order is to infuse 10 μg/kg/min of Dobutrex (dobutamine). If the contents of one 250-mg ampule of Dobutrex are diluted in 250 cc of IV solution, the resulting concentration is 1000 μg/cc. Using a drop factor of 60 gtts/cc, determine the rate in gtts/min. The patient weighs 198 lb.

$$\frac{x \text{ gtts}}{\min \times \text{wt}} = \frac{10 \ \mu g}{\text{kg} \times \min} \times \frac{1 \text{ cc}}{1000 \ \mu g} \times \frac{60 \text{ gtts}}{1 \text{ cc}} \times \frac{1 \text{ kg}}{2.2 \text{ lb}} \times \frac{198 \text{ lb}}{\text{wt}}$$

▶ Answer: 54 gtts/min

3. The order is to infuse Intropin (dopamine) 6 μg/kg/min. The concentration of dopamine is 400 mg per 500 cc of IV solution. Determine the rate of infusion in cc/h for a patient weighing 80 kg.

$$\frac{x \text{ cc}}{\text{h} \times \text{wt}} = \frac{6 \ \mu g}{\text{kg} \times \min} \times \frac{1 \text{ mg}}{1000 \ \mu g} \times \frac{500 \text{ cc}}{400 \text{ mg}} \times \frac{60 \min}{1 \text{ h}} \times \frac{80 \text{ kg}}{\text{wt}}$$

▶ Answer: 36 cc/h

4. The order is to infuse Nipride (nitroprusside) 4 μg/kg/min. The concentration of the solution is 50 mg per 500 ml to produce the equivalent of 100 μg/ml. Determine the rate in cc/h for a patient weighing 55 kg.

$$\frac{x \text{ cc}}{\text{h} \times \text{wt}} = \frac{4 \ \mu g}{\text{kg} \times \min} \times \frac{1 \text{ cc}}{100 \ \mu g} \times \frac{60 \min}{1 \text{ h}} \times \frac{55 \text{ kg}}{\text{wt}}$$

▶ Answer: 132 cc/h

5. The order is to reduce the Nipride drip (nitroprusside) to 0.8 μg/kg/min. The concentration of the solution is 200 μg/cc. Determine the rate in cc/h for a patient weighing 66 kg.

$$\frac{x \text{ cc}}{\text{h} \times \text{wt}} = \frac{0.8 \ \mu g}{\text{kg} \times \min} \times \frac{1 \text{ cc}}{200 \ \mu g} \times \frac{60 \min}{1 \text{ h}} \times \frac{66 \text{ kg}}{\text{wt}}$$

▶ Answer: 16 cc/h

▲ CALCULATION OF DOSAGE (μg/kg/min)

Occasionally it is necessary to calculate the exact dosage of a drug the patient is receiving in micrograms per kilogram per minute. In such cases, the rate of the IV will be known and does not have to be calculated.

Example 11.4: The patient is receiving Intropin (dopamine) at a rate of 30 cc/h. The concentration of the medication is 400 mg in 500 cc of 5% dextrose. How many μg/kg/min is the 55-kg patient receiving?

Step 1: State the problem in equation form.

$$\frac{x \ \mu g}{\text{kg} \times \min} = \frac{30 \text{ cc}}{\text{h} \times \text{wt}}$$

Step 2: Identify the conversion factors needed to convert from cc/h/wt to μg/kg/min. The information needed from the problem to identify the conversion factors is: There are 400 mg per 500 cc of IV fluid; the patient weighs 55 kg.

Four conversion factors are used:

A. Convert from cubic centimeters to milligrams.

$$500 \text{ cc} = 400 \text{ mg}$$

B. Convert from milligrams to micrograms.

$$1 \text{ mg} = 1000 \text{ } \mu\text{g}$$

C. Convert from weight to kilograms.

$$\text{wt} = 55 \text{ kg}$$

D. Convert from hours to minutes.

$$1 \text{ h} = 60 \text{ min}$$

Step 3: Put into the equation the form of each conversion factor that will cancel the unwanted labels and leave only the desired labels on both sides of the equal sign.

$$\frac{x \text{ } \mu\text{g}}{\text{kg} \times \text{min}} = \frac{30 \text{ cc}}{\text{h} \times \text{wt}} \times \frac{400 \text{ mg}}{500 \text{ cc}} \times \frac{1000 \text{ } \mu\text{g}}{1 \text{ mg}} \times \frac{\text{wt}}{55 \text{ kg}} \times \frac{1 \text{ h}}{60 \text{ min}}$$

Step 4: Cancel the labels that appear in both the numerator and the denominator on the same side of the equal sign.

$$\frac{x \text{ } \mu\text{g}}{\text{kg} \times \text{min}} = \frac{30}{1} \times \frac{400}{500} \times \frac{1000 \text{ } \mu\text{g}}{1} \times \frac{1}{55 \text{ kg}} \times \frac{1}{60 \text{ min}}$$

Step 5: Complete the required mathematical operations.

$$\frac{x \text{ } \mu\text{g}}{\text{kg} \times \text{min}} = \frac{7.27 \text{ } \mu\text{g}}{\text{kg} \times \text{min}}$$

Therefore, the patient is receiving a dosage of 7.27 μg/kg/min.

Example 11.5: The patient is receiving Nipride (nitroprusside) at a rate of 30 cc/h. The concentration of the Nipride is 50 mg in 250 cc of IV fluid to give the equivalent of 200 μg per cc. The patient's weight is 143 lb. What dose of Nipride is the patient receiving in μg/kg/min?

Step 1: State the problem in equation form.

$$\frac{x \text{ } \mu\text{g}}{\text{kg} \times \text{min}} = \frac{30 \text{ cc}}{\text{h} \times \text{wt}}$$

Step 2: Identify the conversion factors needed to convert from cc/h/wt to μg/kg/min. The information needed from the problem to identify the conversion factors is: There are 200 μg per 1 cc of IV fluid; the patient weighs 143 lb.

Four conversion factors are used:

A. Convert from cubic centimeters to micrograms.

$$1 \text{ cc} = 200 \text{ } \mu\text{g}$$

B. Convert from weight to pounds.

wt = 143 lb

C. Convert from pounds to kilograms.

2.2 lb = 1 kg

D. Convert from hours to minutes.

1 h = 60 min

Step 3: Put into the equation the form of each conversion factor that will cancel the unwanted labels and leave only the desired labels on both sides of the equal sign.

$$\frac{x\ \mu g}{kg \times min} = \frac{30\ cc}{h \times wt} \times \frac{200\ \mu g}{1\ cc} \times \frac{wt}{143\ lb} \times \frac{2.2\ lb}{1\ kg} \times \frac{1\ h}{60\ min}$$

Step 4: Cancel the labels that appear in both the numerator and the denominator on the same side of the equal sign.

$$\frac{x\ \mu g}{kg \times min} = \frac{30}{1} \times \frac{200\ \mu g}{1} \times \frac{1}{143} \times \frac{2.2}{kg} \times \frac{1}{60\ min}$$

Step 5: Complete the required mathematical operations.

$$\frac{x\ \mu g}{kg \times min} = \frac{1.54\ \mu g}{kg \times min}$$

Therefore, the patient is receiving a dosage of 1.54 μg/kg/min.

Example 11.6: The patient is receiving Dobutrex (dobutamine) at a rate of 18 gtts/min through tubing with a drop factor of 60 gtts/cc. The concentration of the medication is 250 mg in 250 cc of IV fluid. Determine the dosage in μg/kg/min the 80 kg patient is receiving.

Step 1: State the problem in equation form.

$$\frac{x\ \mu g}{kg \times min} = \frac{18\ gtts}{min \times wt}$$

Step 2: Identify the conversion factors needed to convert from gtts/min/wt to μg/kg/min. The information needed from the problem to identify the conversion factors is: There are 250 mg per 250 cc of IV fluid; there are 60 drops per 1 cc; the patient weighs 80 kg.

Four conversion factors are used:

A. Convert from drops to cubic centimeters.

60 gtts = 1 cc

B. Convert from cubic centimeters to milligrams.

250 cc = 250 mg

C. Convert from milligrams to micrograms.

1 mg = 1000 μg

D. Convert from weight to kilograms.

wt = 80 kg

Step 3: Put into the equation the form of each conversion factor that will cancel the unwanted labels and leave only the desired labels on both sides of the equal sign.

$$\frac{x\ \mu g}{kg \times min} = \frac{18\ gtts}{min \times wt} \times \frac{1\ cc}{60\ gtts} \times \frac{250\ mg}{250\ cc} \times \frac{1000\ \mu g}{1\ mg} \times \frac{wt}{80\ kg}$$

Step 4: Cancel the labels that appear in both the numerator and the denominator on the same side of the equal sign.

$$\frac{x\ \mu g}{kg \times min} = \frac{18}{min} \times \frac{1}{60} \times \frac{250}{250} \times \frac{1000\ \mu g}{1} \times \frac{1}{80\ kg}$$

Step 5: Complete the required mathematical operations.

$$\frac{x\ \mu g}{kg \times min} = \frac{3.75\ \mu g}{kg \times min}$$

Therefore, the patient is receiving a dosage of 3.75 μg/kg/min.

▶ SOLVED PRACTICE PROBLEMS

1. The order is to infuse Nipride (nitroprusside) 50 mg in 250 cc of 5% dextrose to keep the diastolic blood pressure below 100 mm Hg. Currently the rate is 20 cc/h. Determine the dosage in μg/kg/min that the 70 kg patient is receiving.

$$\frac{x\ \mu g}{kg \times min} = \frac{20\ cc}{h \times wt} \times \frac{50\ mg}{250\ cc} \times \frac{1000\ \mu g}{1\ mg} \times \frac{wt}{70\ kg} \times \frac{1\ h}{60\ min}$$

▶ Answer: $\frac{0.95\ \mu g}{kg \times min}$

2. A 110 lb patient is receiving Intropin (dopamine) 400 mg/500 cc 5% dextrose at 20 gtts/min through a tubing with a drop factor of 60 gtts/cc. Determine the μg/kg/min the patient is receiving.

$$\frac{x\ \mu g}{kg \times min} = \frac{20\ gtts}{min \times wt} \times \frac{1\ cc}{60\ gtts} \times \frac{400\ mg}{500\ cc} \times \frac{1000\ \mu g}{1\ mg} \times \frac{2.2\ lb}{1\ kg} \times \frac{wt}{110\ lb}$$

▶ Answer: $\frac{5.33\ \mu g}{kg \times min}$

3. A 200 lb patient is receiving Nipride (nitroprusside) 50 mg in 250 cc of IV fluid at a rate of 38 cc/h. Determine the dose of Nipride the patient is receiving in μg/kg/min.

$$\frac{x\ \mu g}{kg \times min} = \frac{38\ cc}{h \times wt} \times \frac{50\ mg}{250\ cc} \times \frac{1000\ \mu g}{1\ mg} \times \frac{wt}{200\ lb} \times \frac{2.2\ lb}{1\ kg} \times \frac{1\ h}{60\ min}$$

▶ Answer: $\frac{1.39\ \mu g}{kg \times min}$

4. A 100 kg patient is receiving Intropin (dopamine) at 30 gtts/min through tubing with a drop factor of 60 gtts/cc. The concentration of the dopamine is 400 mg in 250 cc to give an equivalent of 1600 μg per cc. Determine the dosage in μg/kg/min the patient is receiving.

$$\frac{x\,\mu g}{kg \times min} = \frac{30\ gtts}{min \times wt} \times \frac{1\ cc}{60\ gtts} \times \frac{1600\ \mu g}{1\ cc} \times \frac{wt}{100\ kg}$$

▷ **Answer:** $\dfrac{8\,\mu g}{kg \times min}$

5. The patient is receiving Dobutrex (dobutamine) at a rate of 20 cc/h. The concentration of the medication is 250 mg in 500 cc of IV fluid. Determine the μg/kg/min that the 59 kg patient is receiving.

$$\frac{x\,\mu g}{kg \times min} = \frac{20\ cc}{h \times wt} \times \frac{250\ mg}{500\ cc} \times \frac{1000\ \mu g}{1\ mg} \times \frac{wt}{59\ kg} \times \frac{1\ h}{60\ min}$$

▷ **Answer:** $\dfrac{2.82\,\mu g}{kg \times min}$

CASE STUDIES

▶ Case Eleven

T.C. is a 64-year-old female admitted to the coronary care unit with a diagnosis of severe cardiac decompensation. T.C. weighs 109 lb. Currently she has severe dyspnea and her blood pressure is 80/50 mm Hg. Among her medical orders are: oxygen at 3 L/min; cardiac monitor on V1 continuously; vital signs q15min; pulmonary wedge pressure q1h; hourly output; limit fluid to 1500 cc/24 hours; IV of 250 cc D$_5$W at KVO; start Dobutrex at 5 μg/kg/min.

Dobutrex is sent from the pharmacy in a vial with the following label:

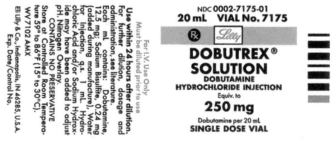

FIGURE 11–1.

The manufacturer's medication insert states that Dobutrex may be reconstituted with 10 ml of sterile water or 5% dextrose. An additional 10 ml of diluent may be added if not completely dissolved. Reconstituted Dobutrex is further diluted to at least 50 ml prior to administration in 5% dextrose, 0.9% sodium chloride, or sodium lactate injection.

Refer to the medication label and the medication insert as needed to answer the following questions.

1. How many kilograms does the patient weigh?
2. What is the minimum amount of IV solution required to dilute one vial of Dobutrex?
3. If one vial of Dobutrex is used to prepare an IV solution using the minimum amount of solution recommended, what will be the concentration (in mg/ml) of the resulting solution?
4. If the decision is made to dissolve the contents of one vial of Dobutrex in a total of 250 ml of IV solution, what will be the concentration (in mg/ml) of the resulting solution?
5. Convert the answer to question 4 from mg/ml to μg/ml.
6. IV administration sets used to administer Dobutrex have what drop factor?
7. How many cc/h are needed to administer the ordered dose of Dobutrex when one vial of medication is dissolved in a total of 250 ml of IV fluid?
8. How many gtts/min are needed to administer the ordered dose of Dobutrex when one vial of medication is dissolved in a total of 250 ml of IV fluid?

For Answers to Case Study Eleven see page 198.

▷ SELF-TEST

1. The order is to give Dobutrex (dobutamine) 250 mg in 250 cc of 5% dextrose at a rate of 6 μg/kg/min. The patient weighs 50 kg. Using 60 gtts/cc, find the rate of the IV in gtts/min and cc/h.
2. The order is to give Intropin (dopamine) at a rate of 7 μg/kg/min. The concentration of the IV solution is 400 μg/ml, with 200 mg dissolved in 500 ml. The patient weighs 130 lb. Find the rate in cc/h.
3. Nipride (nitroprusside) is to be infused at 0.7 μg/kg/min using 50 mg in 250 cc of 5% dextrose. The patient weighs 75 kg. Using 60 gtts/cc, find the rate in cc/h.
4. The order is for Intropin (dopamine) 13 μg/kg/min using 400 mg in 500 cc of normal saline. The patient weighs 90 kg. Using 60 gtts/cc, find the rate in gtts/min.
5. The patient is to receive Nipride at 0.5 μg/kg/min using a concentration of 100 μg/ml. The patient weighs 125 lb. Find the rate in cc/h using 60 gtts/cc.
6. The patient is receiving Intropin (dopamine) at a rate of 25 cc/h. The weight of the patient is 65 kg. The concentration of Intropin is 200 mg in 250 ml. Find the μg/kg/min the patient is receiving.
7. A 180-lb patient is receiving Nipride (nitroprusside) at 30 gtts/min with a drop factor of 60 gtts/cc. The concentration of the solution is 50 mg per 250 cc. Find the μg/kg/min the patient is receiving.
8. A 156-lb patient is receiving Dobutrex (dobutamine) 24 cc/h through a minidrop. The concentration of the solution is 250 mg/250 cc. Find the μg/kg/min that the patient is receiving.

Continued next page

> ▶ **Self-Test Continued**

9. Intropin (dopamine) is being infused at a rate of 35 cc/h using mini-drop tubing. The patient weighs 85 kg and the concentration of the solution is 800 μg/ml. Find the μg/kg/min the patient is receiving.

10. A 78-kg patient is receiving Nipride (nitroprusside) at 20 gtts/min through a minidrop. The concentration of the solution is 200 μg/ml. Find the μg/kg/min the patient is receiving.

For answers to the self-test, see below.

ANSWERS to Case Study Eleven

1. 49.5 kg	4. 1 mg/ml	7. 15 cc/h
2. 50 ml	5. 1000 μg/ml	8. 15 gtts/min
3. 5 mg/ml	6. 60 gtts/cc	

ANSWERS to Self-test

1. 18 gtts/min and 18 cc/h	6. 5.13 μg/kg/min
2. 62 cc/h	7. 1.22 μg/kg/min
3. 16 cc/h	8. 5.64 μg/kg/min
4. 88 gtts/min	9. 5.49 μg/kg/min
5. 17 cc/h	10. 0.85 μg/kg/min

12

Medications Based on Body Surface Area

▲ OBJECTIVES

Upon completion of Chapter 12, the student will be able to:

▶ Correctly calculate the dosage of medications based on body surface area for adults and for children.

▶ Correctly calculate the maximum and minimum amounts of medication for an adult based on the manufacturer's recommendations and the adult's body surface area.

▶ Correctly calculate the maximum and minimum amounts of medication for a child based on the manufacturer's recommendations and the child's body surface area.

▲ DETERMINING BODY SURFACE AREA

Chemotherapeutic drug dosages and pediatric drug dosages may be determined more accurately if they are based on the body surface area (BSA) of the client. Information about the therapeutic dose of a drug based on body surface area is available in the literature accompanying the drug and in the *Physician's Desk Reference (PDR)*.

If the height and weight of a child are known, the BSA may be determined using a nomogram (Figure 12–1). The steps involved in using the nomogram include the following:

1. Find the height of the child in the left-hand column.
2. Find the weight of the child in pounds or kilograms in the right-hand column.
3. Draw a line between the two values.
4. The line where it intersects the column labeled BSA or surface area is the appropriate value.

Example 12.1: A child weighs 52 lb and is 70 in tall. Find the child's BSA using the nomogram.

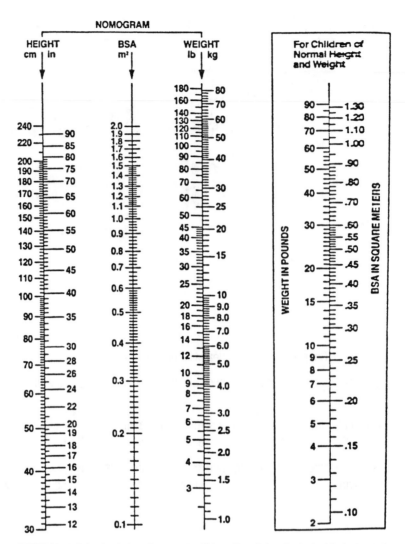

FIGURE 12–1. Estimating body surface area in children. *(From* Nelson Textbook of Pediatrics, *15th Edition. Courtesy W. B. Saunders Co., Philadelphia, PA, with permission.)*

Answer: The BSA value is the point at which the line drawn between 52 lb and 70 in intersects, 1.18 m².

  If you know only the weight of a child who is of normal height, find the child's weight in the enclosed box in Figure 12–1 (second column), then read the corresponding value for the surface area in the same box.

Example 12.2: A child of normal height for his weight weighs 15 lbs. Using the nomogram, what is the value for the child's body surface area?

Answer: 0.36 m²

▲ CALCULATION OF DOSAGE BASED ON BODY SURFACE AREA

After the child's body surface area has been determined, a safe dose for a child may be determined from the adult dose using the following formula:

$$\text{Estimated child dose} = \text{adult dose} \times \frac{\text{child's BSA}}{1.73 \text{ m}^2}$$

Example 12.3: The usual adult dosage for Keflex (cephalexin) is 500 mg PO q6h. The elixir form contains 125 mg/5 cc. Determine the safe dose for the child in Example 12.2. Also determine the number of cc of solution needed to administer the safe dose.

Estimated child dose:

$$x \, mg = 500 \, mg \times \frac{0.36 \, m^2}{1.73 \, m^2}$$

$$x \, mg = 104 \, mg$$

The volume of Keflex needed per dose is:

$$x \, cc = 104 \, mg \times \frac{5 \, cc}{125 \, mg}$$

$$x \, cc = 4.16 \, cc$$

Body surface area (BSA) for an adult may be determined by using the nomogram in Figure 12–2. The same steps are used as those outlined for determining the surface area of a child (see page 199). Body surface area is used for calculating the appropriate dosage of chemotherapeutic drugs for adults.

Example 12.4: An adult weighs 210 lb and is 71 in tall. Find the adult's BSA.

Answer: The BSA value is the point at which the line drawn between 210 lb and 71 in intersects, 2.18 m².

Example 12.5: The order is to give 8000 U/day of asparaginase IV intermittently for 5 days. The adult client weighs 174 lb and is 65 in tall. The therapeutic range for asparaginase is 1000–6000 U/m²/day. Determine the maximum and minimum recommended dose for this client based on BSA. Is the doctor's order within the safe range for the drug?

Part 1
From the nomogram on Figure 12–2, the BSA is 1.89 m².

Part 2

A. Minimum Recommended Daily Dose:

$$\frac{x \, U}{day} = 1.90 \, m^2 \times \frac{1000 \, U}{m^2 \times day}$$

$$\frac{x \, U}{day} = 1900 \, U$$

B. Maximum Recommended Daily Dose:

$$\frac{x \, U}{day} = 1.90 \, m^2 \times \frac{6000 \, U}{m^2 \times day}$$

$$\frac{x \, U}{day} = 11,400 \, U$$

Therefore the doctor's order of 8000 U is within the recommended safe range of 1900 U to 11,400 U.

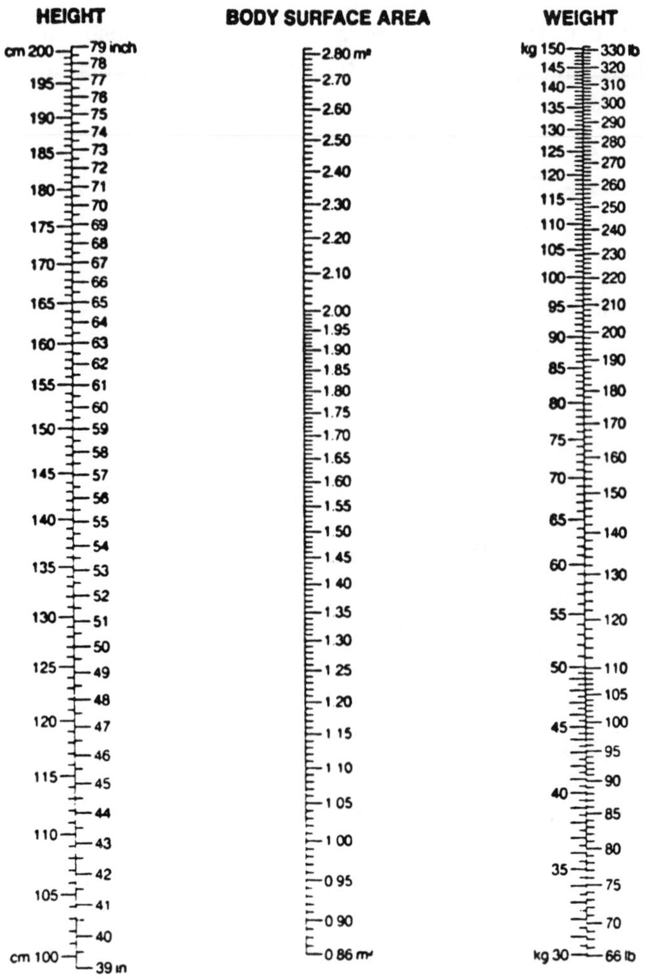

FIGURE 12–2. Estimating body surface area in adults. *(From Lenter C., ed.* Geigy Scientific Tables, *Eighth Edition. Courtesy CIBA-GEIGY, Basle, Switzerland, with permission.)*

► SOLVED PRACTICE PROBLEMS

1. The recommended adult dose of Keflex (cephalexin) is 0.5 to 1 g IM q4–6h. Determine a child's dose whose BSA is 0.23 m². The medication contains 100 mg/cc. Determine the appropriate number of cc.

   A. Minimum Recommended Dose:

   Step 1: $x \, \mathrm{g} = 0.5 \, \mathrm{g} \times \dfrac{0.23 \ \mathrm{m^2}}{1.73 \ \mathrm{m^2}}$

   Step 2: $x \, \mathrm{cc} = 0.07 \, \mathrm{g} \times \dfrac{1000 \ \mathrm{mg}}{1 \ \mathrm{g}} \times \dfrac{1 \ \mathrm{cc}}{100 \ \mathrm{mg}}$

   ► **Answer:** Min = 0.07 g and 0.7 cc

B. Maximum Recommended Dose:

Step 1: $x \, \text{g} = 1 \, \text{g} \times \dfrac{0.23 \, \text{m}^2}{1.73 \, \text{m}^2}$

Step 2: $x \, \text{cc} = 0.13 \, \text{g} \times \dfrac{1000 \, \text{mg}}{1 \, \text{g}} \times \dfrac{1 \, \text{cc}}{100 \, \text{mg}}$

▸ **Answer:** Max = 0.13 g and 1.33 cc

2. The initial adult dose of Decadron (dexamethasone) IM for adults is 4 to 8 mg/day. The solution contains 4 mg/ml. Determine a safe child's dose if the child's BSA is 0.9 m².

Part 1
Minimum Child's Dose:

Step 1: $x \, \text{mg} = 4 \, \text{mg} \times \dfrac{0.9 \, \text{m}^2}{1.73 \, \text{m}^2}$

Step 2: $x \, \text{cc} = 2.1 \, \text{mg} \times \dfrac{1 \, \text{cc}}{4 \, \text{mg}}$

▸ **Answer:** Min = 2.1 mg and 0.53 cc

Part 2
Maximum Child's Dose:

Step 1: $x \, \text{mg} = 8 \, \text{mg} \times \dfrac{0.9 \, \text{m}^2}{1.73 \, \text{m}^2}$

Step 2: $x \, \text{cc} = 4.2 \, \text{mg} \times \dfrac{1 \, \text{cc}}{4 \, \text{mg}}$

▸ **Answer:** Max = 4.2 mg and 1.1 cc

3. The usual adult dose of EES (erythromycin) is 400 mg PO q6h. The liquid form contains 200 mg/5 cc. Determine the equivalent child's dose in mg and cc if the child weighs 28 lb and is of normal height and weight.

Part 1
The BSA is equal to 0.57 m² based on the nomogram.

▸ **Answer:** B.S.A. = 0.57

Part 2
Child's Dose:

Step 1: $x \, \text{mg} = 400 \, \text{mg} \times \dfrac{0.57 \, \text{m}^2}{1.73 \, \text{m}^2}$

Step 2: $x \, \text{cc} = 131.8 \, \text{mg} \times \dfrac{5 \, \text{cc}}{200 \, \text{mg}}$

▸ **Answer:** 131.8 mg and 2.29 cc

4. The order is to give 350 mg of Zovirax (acyclovir) q8h for 5 days to a child who is 65 in tall and weighs 40 lb. Determine the child's BSA and whether the ordered dose is safe. The manufacturer's recommended dose is 250 mg/m^2 for children.

Part 1
The BSA is equal to 0.98 m^2 based on the nomogram.

▷ **Answer:** BSA = 0.98 m^2

Part 2
Recommended Dose:

$$x \text{ mg} = 0.98 \text{ m}^2 \times \frac{250 \text{ mg}}{\text{m}^2}$$

▷ **Answer:** 245 mg Ordered Dose Exceeds Recommended Dose

The doctor's order exceeds the recommended dose. Therefore, verification of the order is necessary prior to administration of the medication.

5. The order is to give 150 mg of Matulane (procarbazine hydrochloride) PO q day for 10 days to an adult. The client's BSA is 1.10 m^2. The manufacturer's recommended dosage range PO is 50–200 mg/m^2/day and not to exceed 300 mg/day. Determine the maximum and minimum recommended doses. Is the doctor's order within the safe range for this drug?

A. Minimum Recommended Daily Dose:

$$\frac{x \text{ mg}}{\text{day}} = 1.10 \text{ m}^2 \times \frac{50 \text{ mg}}{\text{m}^2 \times \text{day}}$$

▷ **Answer:** Min = 55 mg

B. Maximum Recommended Daily Dose:

$$\frac{x \text{ mg}}{\text{day}} = 1.10 \text{ m}^2 \times \frac{200 \text{ mg}}{\text{m}^2 \times \text{day}}$$

▷ **Answer:** Max = 220 mg Does not Exceed Maximum Recommended Dose

The doctor's order of 150 mg does not exceed the maximum recommended daily dose.

▶ **SELF-TEST**

1. According to the manufacturer the therapeutic dose of Gantrisin (sulfisoxazole) for children is 2.25 g/m^2/24 h IV in 4 equal doses. If the child's BSA is 1.4 m^2, determine the total daily dose and the number of mg per dose.
2. The usual adult dose of Demerol (meperidine hydrochloride) is 75 mg q4h. If a child's BSA is 1.3 m^2, determine the child's safe dose.

Continued next page

▶ **Self-Test Continued**

3. The usual adult dose of EES (erythromycin) is 400 mg PO q6h. The liquid form contains 200 mg per 5 cc. Determine the equivalent child's dose in mg and cc if the child is 120 cm tall and weighs 25 kg.

4. The usual adult dose of Solu-Medrol (hydrocortisone) is 100 mg. Determine a child's dose in mg and cc if the child's BSA is 0.7 m^2.

5. A usual adult dose of Terramycin (oxytetracycline) is 100 mg IM q8h. The drug is available in solution of 100 mg per 2 cc. If the child is 70 cm tall and weighs 8 kg, determine a child's dose in mg and cc.

6. The order is to give Cisplatin 200 mg IV qd for 5 days. The manufacturer's recommended dose for ovarian cancer is 50–100 mg/m^2/day IV for adults. The adult client is 150 cm tall and weighs 95 kg. Determine the maximum and minimum recommended doses. Is the ordered dose a safe dose?

7. Determine the recommended dose of Matulane (procarbazine hydrochloride) for a child whose BSA is 1.4 m^2. The manufacturer's recommended child's PO dose is 100 mg/m^2/day.

8. The order is to give 220 mg of Cytosar-U (cytarabine) to an adult who is 135 cm tall and weighs 150 lb. The recommended dose range is 100–150 mg/m^2/day in continuous IV. Determine if the dose is within recommended values.

9. The order is to give 60 mg of BICNU (carmustine) per day per IV to a child whose BSA is 0.8 m^2. The recommended range for a child is 75–100 mg/m^2/day per IV. Determine if the dose is within the recommended values.

10. Determine the maximum and minimum recommended doses of Matulane (procarbazine hydrochloride) for an adult whose BSA is 1.95 m^2. The recommended dose range is 50–200 mg/m^2/day for 10–20 days.

For answers to the self-test, see below.

1. 3150 mg/day and 787.5 mg/dose
2. 56.36 mg
3. 208.1 mg and 5.2 cc
4. 40.46 mg and 0.81 cc
5. 23.7 mg and 0.47 cc
6. Min = 92.5 and Max = 185 mg per day
   Ordered dose *exceeds* recommended dose.
7. 140 mg per day
8. Min = 150 mg and Max = 225 mg per day
   Ordered dose *does not* exceed recommended dose.
9. Min = 60 mg and Max = 80 mg per day
   Ordered dose *does not* exceed recommended dose.
10. Min = 97.5 mg and Max = 390 mg per day

Common Abbreviations and Symbols Related to Medication Administration

ABBREVIATION	MEANING	ABBREVIATION	MEANING
a	before	elix	elixir
aa	of each	et (&)	and
ac	before meals	ext	extract
ad	up to		
ad lib	as desired	F, ºF	Fahrenheit
amp	ampule	fl dr, $\mathfrak{z}$	fluid dram
aq	water		
		Gm, g, gm	gram
b.i.d., B.I.D.	two times a day	gr	grain
BP	blood pressure	gtt	drop
		h, hr	hour
c, c̄	with	H	hypodermic
C, ºC	centigrade; Celsius	h.s.	hour of sleep; bedtime
cc	cubic centimeter	in	inch
caps	capsule	IM	intramuscular
comp	compound	IV	intravascular
CVP	central venous pressure	IVP	intravenous push
		IVPB	intravenous piggyback
d	day		
DC	discontinue	K, kg	kilogram
dr	dram	KVO	keep vein open

ABBREVIATION	MEANING	ABBREVIATION	MEANING
L	liter	R	rectal; respiration
lb	pound	rep	repeat
μg, mcg	microgram	$\bar{s}$	without
mEq	milliequivalent	SC, sc, subq, SQ	subcutaneously
mg	milligram	SL	beneath the tongue
m, m_x	minim		
min	minute	sos	once only if needed
ml	milliliter		
mU	milliunit	sol	solution
		sp	spirits
n, noct	night	$\overline{ss}$, ss	one-half
no (#)	number	stat	immediately
NPO	nothing by mouth	supp	suppository
		susp	suspension
OD	right eye	syr	syrup
os	mouth		
OS	left eye	t, tsp	teaspoon
OU	in each eye	T	temperature; tablespoon
oz, ℥	ounce		
		tab	tablet
P	pulse	TBA	to be absorbed
PO, po	by mouth	tbsp, T	tablespoon
pc	after meals	t.i.d., T.I.D.	three times a day
per	through or by	TKO	to keep open
pre-op	before surgery	TPN	total parenteral nutrition
prn	as needed or required	tr, tinct	tincture
		troch	lozenges
pulv	powder		
		U, u	unit
q	each, every	ung	ointment
qd	every day	UO	urinary output
qh	every hour		
q2h, q2hr	every two hours	via	by way of
q3h, q3hr	every three hours		
q.i.d., QID	four times a day	wt	weight
q.o.d.	every other day		
qs	as much as required; sufficient amount	X, x	multiplied by
		%	percent

NUMBERS USED IN APOTHECARY SYSTEM

I, i	= one	IX, ix	= nine
II, ii	= two	X, x	= ten
III, iii	= three	ss	$= \frac{1}{2}$
IV, iv	= four	iss	$= 1\frac{1}{2}$
V, v	= five	iiss	$= 2\frac{1}{2}$
VI, vi	= six	iiiss	$= 3\frac{1}{2}$
VII, vii	= seven	ivss	$= 4\frac{1}{2}$
VIII, viii	= eight		

Calculations with Percent Solutions

B

Solutions used for therapeutic purposes are made by dissolving a substance called a solute in a liquid medium called a solvent. The resulting solutions have a composition that can be expressed on the basis of the amount of solute added to 100 milliliters of solution.

1. Adding 5 grams of sodium chloride to enough water to make 100 milliliters of solution yields a 5% solution.
2. Adding 50 milliliters of alcohol to enough water to make 100 milliliters of solution yields a 50% solution.
3. A 5% dextrose IV solution is made by adding enough dextrose to 1 liter to make it equal to 5 grams per 100 milliliters.
4. A 0.9% sodium chloride solution is made by adding enough sodium chloride to 1 liter to make it equal to 0.9 grams per 100 milliliters.

As can be noted from the four examples above, when the solute added is a solid, the percent solution is based on the number of grams of solute added to 100 milliliters of solution. When the solute is a liquid, the percent is calculated on the number of milliliters added to 100 milliliters of the solution.

Additional applications of the concepts related to percent solutions are illustrated in the three examples given below.

Example B.1: Determine how many grams of glucose are contained in 1 liter of 5% glucose solution.

Known: 1 L = 1000 ml
         5% means 5 g per 100 ml of solution

Then:

$$x \text{ g} = 1000 \text{ ml} \times \frac{5 \text{ g}}{100 \text{ ml}}$$

$$x \text{ g} = 50 \text{ g}$$

Example B.2: Determine how many grams of sodium chloride are contained in 1 liter of 0.9% sodium chloride.

Known: 1 L = 1000 ml

0.9% means 0.9 g per 100 ml of solution

Then:

$$x\,\text{g} = 1000\,\text{ml} \times \frac{0.9\,\text{g}}{100\,\text{ml}}$$

$$x\,\text{g} = 9\,\text{g}$$

Example B.3: An IV solution contains dextrose 50%. How many grams of dextrose are contained in 500 milliliters of this IV solution?

Known: 50% means 50 g per 100 ml

Then:

$$x\,\text{g} = 500\,\text{ml} \times \frac{50\,\text{g}}{100\,\text{ml}}$$

$$x\,\text{g} = 250\,\text{g}$$

Temperature Conversions

There are two different temperature scales in common use today. The familiar Fahrenheit scale places normal body temperature at 98.6 degrees. The Celsius, or Centigrade, scale places normal body temperature at 37 degrees.

The Fahrenheit temperature scale is the scale most commonly used in the health sciences. The Celsius, or Centigrade, scale is the scale of choice in many other scientific fields. Some health professionals and some health institutions use the Celsius scale in preference to the Fahrenheit scale. It is, therefore, occasionally necessary to carry out conversions between the two temperature scales.

Conversions between the two temperature scales cannot be accomplished by dimensional analysis. This is due to the fact that the two scales are not directly proportional to each other. Dimensional analysis is applicable only to conversion among units that are directly proportional to each other. Therefore, temperature conversions must be accomplished by means of memorized formulas.

▲ CONVERTING FROM CELSIUS TO FAHRENHEIT

The formula required is: $F = (9/5 \times C) + 32$

Example C.1: Convert 40° Celsius to the equivalent Fahrenheit degrees.

$F = (9/5 \times C) + 32$
$F = (9/5 \times 40) + 32$
$F = 72 + 32$
$F = 104$

Therefore, 40C is equal to 104F.

Example C.2: Convert 38.3° Celsius to the equivalent Fahrenheit degrees.

$F = (9/5 \times C) + 32$
$F = (9/5 \times 38.3) + 32$
$F = 68.94 + 32$
$F = 100.94$, may be rounded to 100.9

Therefore, 38.3C is equal to 100.9F.

▲ CONVERTING FROM FAHRENHEIT TO CELSIUS

The formula required is: $C = 5/9(F - 32)$

Example C.3: Convert 99.6º Fahrenheit to the equivalent Celsius degrees.

$C = 5/9(F - 32)$
$C = 5/9(99.6 - 32)$
$C = 5/9(67.60)$
$C = 37.56$, may be rounded to 37.6

Therefore, 99.6F is equal to 37.6C.

Example C.4: Convert 100.5º Fahrenheit to the equivalent Celsius degrees.

$C = 5/9(F - 32)$
$C = 5/9(100.5 - 32)$
$C = 5/9(68.5)$
$C = 38.05$, may be rounded to 38.1

Therefore, 100.5F is equal to 38.1C.

Index

LICENSE AGREEMENT AND LIMITED WARRANTY

READ THE FOLLOWING TERMS AND CONDITIONS CAREFULLY BEFORE OPENING THIS DISK PACKAGE. THIS IS AN AGREEMENT BETWEEN YOU AND APPLETON & LANGE (THE "COMPANY"). BY OPENING THIS SEALED PACKAGE, YOU ARE AGREEING TO BE BOUND BY THESE TERMS AND CONDITIONS. IF YOU DO NOT AGREE WITH THESE TERMS AND CONDITIONS, DO NOT OPEN THE DISK PACKAGE. PROMPTLY RETURN THE DISK PACKAGE AND ALL ACCOMPANYING ITEMS TO THE COMPANY.

1. GRANT OF LICENSE: In consideration of your adoption of textbooks and/or other materials published by the Company, and your agreement to abide by the terms and conditions of this Agreement, the Company grants to you a nonexclusive right to use and display the copy of the enclosed software program (hereinafter the "SOFTWARE") so long as you comply with the terms of this Agreement. The Company reserves all rights not expressly granted to you under this Agreement. This license is *not* a sale of the original SOFTWARE or any copy to you.

2. USE RESTRICTIONS: You may *not* sell, license, transfer or distribute copies of the SOFTWARE or Documentation to others. You may *not* reverse engineer, disassemble, decompile, modify, adapt, translate or otherwise reproduce the SOFTWARE or any part of it, or create derivative works based on the SOFTWARE or the Documentation without the prior written consent of the Company.

3. MISCELLANEOUS: This Agreement shall be construed in accordance with the laws of the United States of America and the State of New York, except for that body of law dealing with conflicts of law, and shall benefit the Company, its affiliates and assignees. If any provision of this Agreement is found void or unenforceable, the remainder will remain valid and enforceable according to its terms. Use, duplication or disclosure of the SOFTWARE by the U.S. Government is subject to the restricted rights applicable to commercial computer software under FAR 52.227.19 and DFARS 252.277-7013.

4. LIMITED WARRANTY AND DISCLAIMER OF WARRANTY: Because this SOFTWARE is being given to you without charge, the Company makes no warranties about the SOFTWARE, which is provided "AS-IS." **THE COMPANY DISCLAIMS ALL WARRANTIES, EXPRESS OR IMPLIED, INCLUDING WITHOUT LIMITATION, THE IMPLIED WARRANTIES OF MERCHANTABILITY AND FITNESS FOR A PARTICULAR PURPOSE. THE COMPANY DOES NOT WARRANT, GUARANTEE OR MAKE ANY REPRESENTATION REGARDING THE USE OR THE RESULTS OF THE USE OF THE SOFTWARE. IN NO EVENT, SHALL THE COMPANY, ITS PARENTS SUBSIDIARIES, AFFILIATES, LICENSORS, DIRECTORS, OFFICERS, EMPLOYEES, AGENTS, SUPPLIERS OR CONTRACTORS BE LIABLE FOR ANY INCIDENTAL, INDIRECT, SPECIAL OR CONSEQUENTIAL DAMAGES ARISING OUT OF OR IN CONNECTION WITH THE LICENSE GRANTED UNDER THIS AGREEMENT INCLUDING, WITHOUT LIMITATION, LOSS OF USE, LOSS OF DATA, LOSS OF INCOME OR PROFIT, OR OTHER LOSSES SUSTAINED AS A RESULT OF INJURY TO ANY PERSON, OR LOSS OF OR DAMAGE TO PROPERTY, OR CLAIMS OF THIRD PARTIES, EVEN IF THE COMPANY OR AN AUTHORIZED REPRESENTATIVE OF THE COMPANY HAS BEEN ADVISED OF THE POSSIBILITY OF SUCH DAMAGES.**

SOME JURISDICTIONS DO NOT ALLOW THE EXCLUSION OF IMPLIED WARRANTIES OR THE LIMITATION ON LIABILITY FOR INCIDENTAL, INDIRECT, SPECIAL OR CONSEQUENTIAL DAMAGES, SO THE ABOVE LIMITATIONS MAY NOT ALWAYS APPLY. THE WARRANTIES IN THIS AGREEMENT GIVE YOU SPECIFIC LEGAL RIGHTS AND YOU MAY ALSO HAVE OTHER RIGHTS WHICH VARY IN ACCORDANCE WITH LOCAL LAW.

No sales personnel or other representative of any party involved in the distribution of the software is authorized by the Company to make any warranties with respect to the software beyond what is contained in this agreement. Oral statements do not constitute warranties, shall not be relied upon by you and are not part of this agreement. The entire agreement between you and the Company is embodied therein.

ACKNOWLEDGMENT

YOU ACKNOWLEDGE THAT YOU HAVE READ THIS AGREEMENT, UNDERSTAND IT AND AGREE TO BE BOUND BY ITS TERMS AND CONDITIONS, YOU ALSO AGREE THAT THIS AGREEMENT IS THE COMPLETE AND EXCLUSIVE AGREEMENT BETWEEN YOU AND THE COMPANY.

Should you have any questions concerning this agreement or if you wish to contact the Company for any reason, please contact in writing: Simon & Schuster, c/o Starpack, 237 22nd Street, Greeley, CO 80631.   (800) 991-0077

Unicalc will signal the end of a session by sounding a series of beeps after every question in either session has been answered. To continue studying, simply exit the session and begin again.